"Finally, a comprehensive anger workbook for women—thoughtful and informative, this book is a must for any woman who struggles with constructively expressing anger. Petracek has created a thoughtful and informative guide that offers insight into the specific difficulties women have with anger. This workbook is full of examples and exercises that will help the reader identify how she currently manages her anger, how stress and self-esteem relate to anger, and ways to appropriately express anger and improve relationships. This exceptional book will help women stop destructive patterns of anger, whether they lash out or hold it in, and have healthier, happier lives and relationships. I am thrilled to have such a great resource for my clients."

—Vallerie E. Coleman, Ph.D., psychologist and adjunct faculty member in the Department of Psychology at Loyola Marymount University

"Petracek uses a commonsense, realistic approach to helping women deal with their anger. I found a wealth of information on the pages of this book; it is an excellent tool for women whether they have mild or major challenges with rage. Petracek takes the mind, body, and spirit into account when teaching women how to channel their anger in a healthy way."

—Jan Brown, executive director of the Domestic Abuse Helpline for Men

"A much-needed book. The problem of women's anger is often minimized in our society, but not by Petracek who, thankfully, takes this subject seriously. Having worked for many years with angry and aggressive women, she offers some practical and innovative solutions. I especially enjoyed her sections on anger-ins vs. anger-outs and the chapter on parenting."

—John Hamel, LCSW, author of *High Conflict to Battering* and director of John Hamel & Associates, a counseling firm in San Raphael, CA

"A much-needed, long-awaited book on the subject."

—Ruth Gottstein, publisher of Volcano Press

THE·ANGER WORKBOOK FOR·WOMEN

How to Keep Your Anger
from Undermining
Your Self-Esteem,
Your Emotional Balance,
and Your Relationships

Laura J. Petracek, Ph.D., LCSW

Foreword by Sandra P. Thomas, Ph.D., RN, FAAN

New Harbinger Publications, Inc.

This book is dedicated in memory of my mother, Carole. Thank you for believing in me.

To my daughter, Lena Rose. I believed in you long before you were ever conceived, and I will believe in you long past the end of all eternity.

And to all of my clients in the W.O.V.E.N. groups. Thank you for sharing your experience, strength, and hope and allowing your stories to be shared with other women who still struggle with their anger.

Contents

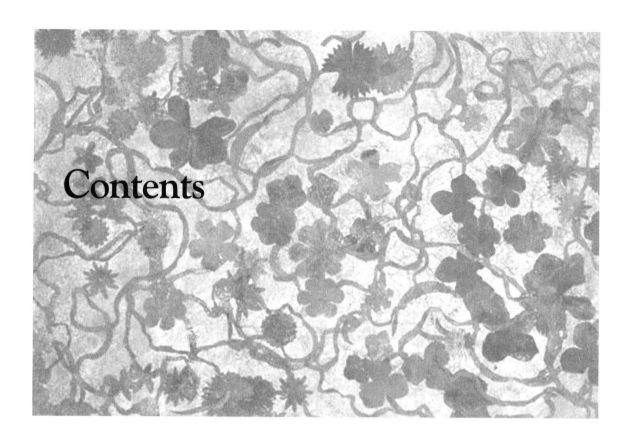

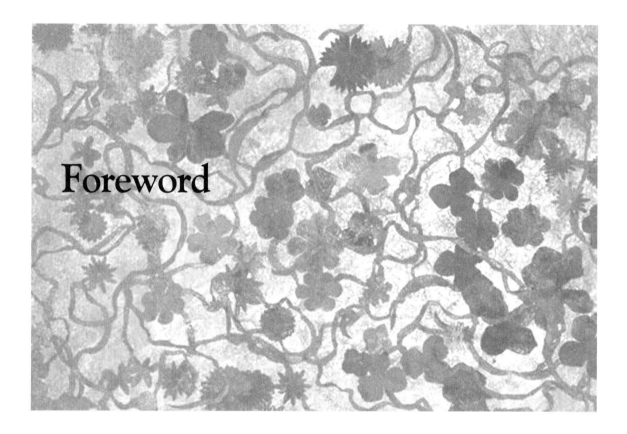

Foreword

I AM delighted to offer a few thoughts about women's anger as a prelude to this excellent anger workbook for women. We have come a long way since Harriet Lerner, author of *The Dance of Anger* (1985), labeled women's anger a "taboo topic." Taboo it certainly was while I was growing up in the South, where women used euphemisms when angry ("I'm a little upset") instead of forthrightly claiming their angry feelings. Anger was taboo because women feared they would be viewed as unfeminine. They feared alienating their significant others. They did not wish to disrupt the status quo. And so their anger went underground, festering inside—and occasionally surfacing in indirect manifestations such as backbiting or gossiping.

Women's roles have undergone a sea change since I was growing up. Women have successfully pursued a host of nontraditional career options, and they have even made gains in pay equity. The glass ceiling is being shattered in boardrooms across the land.

It would seem logical to presume that contemporary "liberated" women would have no difficulty expressing their anger. But I have been conducting research on women for fifteen years, and over and over—whether I am studying white or black women, rural or urban women, CEOs or nurses or teachers or social workers—I hear women describe their sense of powerlessness regarding anger-provoking behaviors of spouses, friends, and coworkers. They want someone or something to change, but they cannot seem to make the desired change happen. Whether they seethe in silence or scream and shout, women do not feel good about how they handle anger.

Their anger is complex because it is intertwined with hurt. Women often say, "I don't know whether I am angry or hurt." They had expected certain behaviors from their spouses, friends, and coworkers—behaviors of respect, consideration, fairness, responsibility, truthfulness, reciprocity. Disillusionment mingles with the anger of unmet expectations. Because there is no resolution of the anger-provoking issue, women often ruminate about an injustice for quite a long time.

Women must learn healthier ways to manage anger. This book is devoted to helping women learn and practice new anger behaviors. Mismanaged anger has been implicated in depression, high blood pressure, migraine headaches, obesity, substance abuse, and many other conditions. Effective anger management skills facilitate not only improved intimate relationships but also improved physical and mental health. In this book, you will find out how to assess your behavioral, cognitive, and physiological anger. You will learn about anger's connections to stress and self-esteem. You will learn to use your anger constructively.

You are embarking on a journey of self-discovery and emotional growth. Dr. Laura Petracek will be your steadfast companion on this journey. I wish you Godspeed.

—Sandra P. Thomas, Ph.D., RN, FAAN

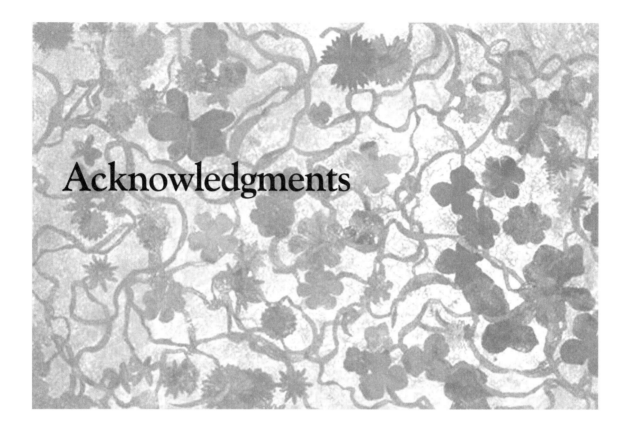

Acknowledgments

I AM deeply appreciative of everyone who has supported me during the process of writing this workbook. In particular, I want to express my gratitude to my family and friends, especially Margot, Sandy, Tamara, and my sister Therese. I am grateful to my acquisitions editor, Tesilya Hanauer, for her belief in this workbook and guidance throughout the process, and my copyeditor, Jessica Beebe, for her corrections and suggestions. I want to especially thank my niece Molly for her wonderful, expressive drawings of women's emotions and my sister Celia for lending her time and expertise on art therapy. I want to extend my gratitude to my colleagues in the field of anger management, Valerie Coleman, Brenda Shook, David Fontes, Sandra Thomas, Darlene Pratt, Charles Spielberger, and John Hamel, for reading drafts of various chapters and providing their expertise and feedback. I am indebted to Roland Maiuro, whose suggestion to conduct my dissertation study on women and anger eventually led me to write this book. I want to also thank Tamara and Marion, who spent endless hours helping me organize the material and typed and retyped the manuscript. I would also like to acknowledge the women in the W.O.V.E.N. groups who were my teachers as much as I was theirs. By sharing their anger experiences, they provided the foundation of this workbook. I want to express my profound gratitude to all of these people. Finally, I want to thank my higher power, whom I choose to call God, for giving me a spiritual wake-up call to accomplish my dream of writing this book.

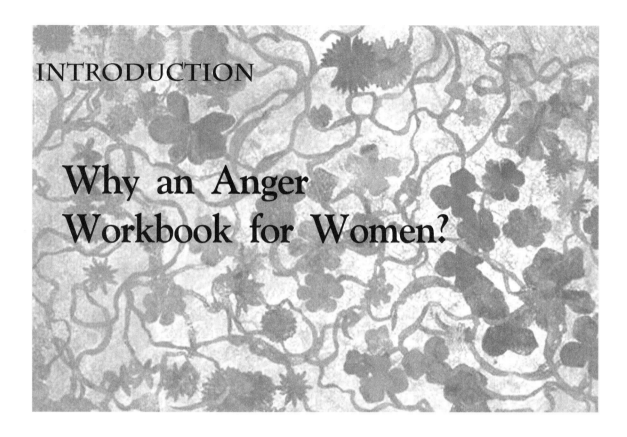

INTRODUCTION

Why an Anger Workbook for Women?

ANGER IS anger, whether men express it or women express it, right? Get real! Men and women express anger much differently. And, if a woman picked up a typical anger management workbook, she would soon find that it was written for men. This exclusive focus stems from our societal beliefs that women don't have anger control problems. Women are raised to be caregivers and to be nurturing and loving. Women are seen as victims—and undeniably, women often are victims.

As a therapist who treats primarily women, I've found an increasing number of women are seeking help for their anger problems. In 1993, while I was a doctoral intern at Harborview Hospital's anger management program in Seattle, Washington, I couldn't help but be amazed at the number of women seeking help for anger issues. At the suggestion of my supervisor, Roland Maiuro, I started my first anger group specifically designed for women, which later became the basis for my doctoral dissertation. My years of research, group facilitation, and working with women one-on-one have guided me in developing this interactive workbook exclusively for women.

Anger-In versus Anger-Out

Most women in our society are either not in touch with their anger or feel their anger but don't know how to express it. Lisa's story is a good example of not expressing anger.

One day I was driving down Masonic Street looking for parking. I saw a spot and put on my signal to let the other drivers know I was backing into the parking space. No one would give me the right of way. Finally, when the cars stopped coming, I proceeded to park my car. Out of nowhere, I saw a car that must have been speeding about sixty to seventy miles an hour coming right at me. The driver almost rear-ended me. She was blowing her horn, yelling out her window calling me names, and flipped me off. In that moment I became very angry but didn't know what to do with it, so I just wished she would run into something and die. I couldn't shake the feeling for the rest of the day.

Lisa's expression of anger is what Sandra Thomas (1993) and Charles Spielberger (1995) call *anger-in*. This is the type of anger most women experience. Anger-in involves keeping angry feelings to yourself. Women who fall into this category try to act as if everything is okay—as if nothing happened. This is the unfortunate result of the way women are socialized to believe that outward expression of anger is unladylike, antimaternal, and sexually unattractive. Women who outwardly express anger are often considered unfeminine or called shrews, bitches, man-haters, and other not-so-nice names. And what woman wants that? Instead, women direct their anger at themselves by overeating, becoming depressed, and hurting themselves. If you are woman who primarily keeps your anger in, your goal in this workbook will be to learn how to be more assertive.

Anger-out (Thomas 1993) involves expressing anger by venting your rage at another person, or attacking or blaming another person, possibly to the point of pushing, shoving, or kicking that person.

One afternoon Kristin made an appointment with me to seek help with her anger-out expression.

One day I was crossing the street, coming from the beach, and there was bumper-to-bumper traffic. A man motioned for me to cross the street. He said with a sneer, "But hurry up! I am trying to follow someone." In a calm voice and with a sarcastic smile, I said, "Okay, but I really don't think it's going to be a problem," because the traffic was not budging. His reply was loud and angry: "Shut up, you f—ing bitch!" I thought I was going to instantly combust, and turned to go after him. I had my skateboard in hand, threatening him with it, shouting obscenities back at him as I approached his car. The traffic began to move and I stopped in my tracks and turned away. I was feeling no release, and I was upset with the idea that I had to sit with my intense anger. I also felt guilty, remorseful, and embarrassed by how I had acted. The zero-to-sixty my emotions went through was the most intense rush of adrenaline I have ever felt.

Women who express anger-out behavior usually feel they do not have any control over their anger. They are also the ones most often referred to participate in an anger management group. If you are a woman who has trouble keeping a lid on your anger, this workbook will help you learn assertiveness skills along with coping skills to keep your anger in check.

Men versus Women

The methods and interventions of anger control I have developed throughout my years of counseling women are different than those used for men. Teaching cognitive behavioral skills is the primary method of intervention in traditional anger workbooks for men. However, women are much more relational; therefore, interactive techniques are the primary method of intervention. In fact, women do particularly well in group therapy settings. Men are challenged to stop abusing power and to learn to share power equally with their partners. On the other hand, women are challenged to understand the negative cultural view of the direct communication of their anger. Women must recognize their anger as legitimate and allow themselves to express it appropriately.

What This Book Offers You

This workbook is broken down into chapters that deal with specific issues influencing your anger. Included are some simple but important exercises to assist you as you continue on your learning journey. In the first chapter, you will learn how women's socialization affects their anger. You will also begin the process of understanding how you express your anger.

In chapter 2 you'll explore the world of feelings. You will learn to name your feelings and recognize how these feelings can affect your expression of anger.

In chapter 3 you'll learn about different types of anger. Determining which type of anger you have, either anger-in or anger-out, will help you identify the best approach to dealing with your anger. In chapter 4 we'll discuss the impact of boundaries on anger. Many women with anger control issues also have difficulties setting boundaries or being aware of other people's boundaries.

Stress, lowered self-esteem, and anger usually come hand in hand. In chapter 5 you will identify your stressors and self-esteem issues and see how they connect to your anger. I have included some relaxation techniques and exercises to build your self-esteem.

As you move into chapter 6, you will work on your anger as it relates to children. The most obvious impact is the possibility of physical and emotional trauma inflicted on children. But your anger habit can have an impact that you are not aware of. Having multiple responsibilities of raising children, working, and taking care of a home can create stress that leads to anger outbursts. Your children pick up on the way you express anger and use it as a guide for expressing their own anger, the same way they mimic your other habits.

Many of the negative feelings that contribute to your anger probably originated from your own childhood. In chapter 7 you will be asked to dig into your childhood, where you can begin to recognize what messages you may have received. Childhood experiences can be gruesome on many levels. From your family of origin to your schoolmates, your childhood experiences have placed barriers for you to break through. Someone once said to me, "Childhood is what you spend the rest of your life trying to get over!"

As you begin to understand your anger, the next step is to develop skills and tools for better communication. In chapter 8 you will learn about various styles of communication. Using I-statements and time-outs are just two of many effective skills necessary for direct and respectful communication. Along with learning those skills, you will explore constructive problem solving necessary to express your anger in a positive way.

In chapter 9 you'll learn about self-talk. We all do it—but it's the particular words we use that can bring us down quickly. Chances are you've done a lot of self-talk in your life without even being aware of it. This chapter deals specifically with the impact of positive and negative self-talk.

Chapter 10 covers the effects of anger on your physical health. There are also some mood disorders associated with anger problems; chapter 11 addresses three predominant mood disorders: premenstrual syndrome, depression, and bipolar disorder. Assessments are included to help you determine if you show signs of a mood disorder. In chapter 12 you will tackle the effects of alcohol on your anger. If you have an alcohol use problem, it may be crucial that you deal with it first, as this could be your biggest trigger for anger.

Being able to forgive is an important part of healing. In chapter 13 you will see how spirituality can be a great tool for healing anger. Now, *spiritual* is not the same as *religious*. Spirituality means connecting with a power greater than yourself, whatever you choose to call it. Having anger control issues can zap the energy out of your life because you feel lonely, depressed, and without purpose. Spirituality gives purpose, hope, and love in our lives. Reconnecting with your spirituality can provide you with some peace and help put minor aggravations in perspective.

Whether you have difficulty expressing your anger or keeping your anger in control, this workbook offers a new clinical map of action. Some additional skills offered in this workbook are

* developing a sense of yourself separate from others,

* building better boundaries,

* developing a social support system,

* working out your anger and rage issues regarding your family of origin,

* responding to your anger in a more effective and positive way,

* using your head when you're feeling anger,

* identifying your anger triggers,

* increasing your awareness of anger and your feelings,

* learning self-care skills,

* working through your guilt response to anger, and

* responding effectively to the reactions of others.

Your Journey Begins

Anger is one of many emotions we experience. It's neither good nor bad; it just is. You can get free of your anger if you choose to take action and make the changes suggested in this workbook. Anger can be a healthy motivator. Because women are not as comfortable with anger, it can become overwhelming. When you deny your anger, it doesn't go away. You can learn to enjoy your anger by taking the positive action it nudges you to do.

Although this workbook suggests a variety of techniques drawn from the very best social, psychological, medical, and spiritual literature, it is not a substitute for seeking professional psychotherapy or joining a women's anger therapy group. It is a road map for exploring your anger and other emotions through journaling, questionnaires, and art and music therapy exercises. You may decide while you're working through the workbook to seek professional help. Look for a therapist who's right for you, preferably a woman therapist who is experienced with anger issues.

Most women have never had the opportunity or encouragement to really experience their anger. By trying different assertive behaviors when experiencing anger, you will soon learn how to work with your anger in a positive way. Being a woman with anger issues is a difficult task, considering how women have been taught for most of their lives to deny their anger. This is not to say anger is bad. On the contrary, anger can be a very useful emotion. It can be used to generate energy that can ultimately help us keep our power. Together, we as women can journey toward wholeness and healing. You will soon learn how to be the woman you were meant to be.

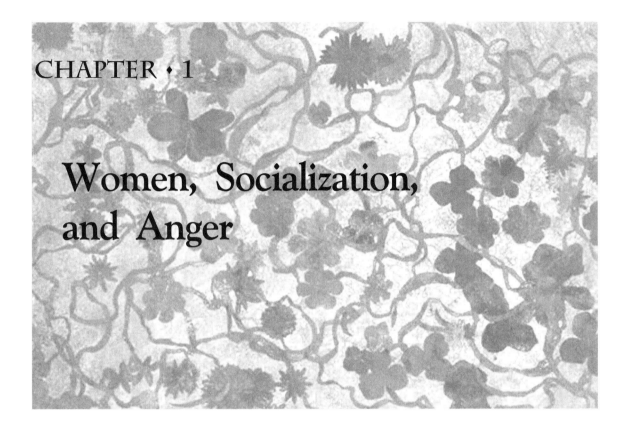

CHAPTER · 1

Women, Socialization, and Anger

WOMEN AND men are socialized in different ways about how they express anger and aggression. Women have been discouraged from the awareness and expression of anger. From an early age, women are taught that expressing anger is unacceptable to others and will lead to negative consequences such as being abandoned or having affection withheld. Just because you have blocks to expressing anger does not mean that you are not angry. It is the anger you do not express that can do the most damage to you and to your relationships with other people. Unfortunately, many women go overboard in controlling negative feelings; they control not only their expression but also their awareness of anger.

Girls have been encouraged to keep their anger down; they are not encouraged to act out anger in a physical way. Women's anger, therefore, is often misdirected in passive-aggressive ways such as sulking, backstabbing, malicious gossip, and writing someone off and never speaking to that person again. Women usually get the message that anger is unpleasant and unfeminine. According to Tangney and colleagues (1992), women generally have less trouble with anger than men do because women manage it better. Women are not as aggressive as men in expressing anger and tend to talk out their anger more. Women are more proactive and use more problem-solving approaches in discussing problems.

Many times our first thought or feeling about a situation is a conditioned response; our socialized response; what we think society, our family, our friends, or our partner would want us to say, think, or feel. The following exercise shows how if we review a situation after it has occurred, we give ourselves time to examine how we truly feel about the situation.

How do you see yourself? Cut a picture that represents you out of a popular magazine. Choose any magazine and any picture. Glue or tape the picture here.

Now do some free association with this picture. Write down your feelings about what you see and what you feel.

. . . .

. . . .

. . . .

. . . .

. . . .

. . . .

. . . .

Wait until the next day or, if you are using this book with a group, the next group session.

Now analyze what you think you were really experiencing and feeling when you picked out that picture.

. . . .

. . . .

. . . .

. . . .

. . . .

. . . .

. . . .

. . . .

. . . .

❖

Indirect Ways of Expressing Anger (Anger-In)

According to a research study by DiGiuseppe and Tafrate (forthcoming), women are more likely to be angry longer, more likely to be resentful, and less likely to express their anger compared to men. Most women are very creative about finding indirect ways of expressing their anger. Because most women learned to suppress their anger, it often is expressed in unhealthy ways. Remember the last time you did a slow burn at home or gave your partner the cold shoulder? Do you think he or she got the message that you were angry?

Many women were taught as children that anger is not a "good" emotion to express. Mothers are more likely to allow anger expression for their sons than for their daughters (Cox, Stabb, and Bruckner 1999). An example of this social conditioning comes from Tami, who described a typical childhood scene.

> My brother and I were playing with Legos, and we kept bickering over certain pieces. My brother grabbed a handful of Legos and threw them at me. My mother scolded him and said, "Stop throwing stuff at your sister!" We stopped arguing briefly and went back to building our projects. But I was stewing inside because he just messed up what I was working on. Finally, I just burst out, "Now mine is all messed up!" and threw the Legos at him. I spent the next forty-five minutes in a chair with my hands neatly folded in my lap while I received a lecture about proper behavior for girls.

Tami and her brother were obviously taught different lessons about handling anger, and they learned that rules about anger apply differently to boys than girls.

Since women are not encouraged to express anger directly, they learn to express it indirectly instead. This is anger-in. Here are some ways women express anger indirectly.

BLAMING: Name-calling, put-downs, not taking responsibility. Saying *You did this.*

SARCASM: Mean and hostile joking at someone else's expense.

VINDICTIVENESS: Taking action so that you do not feel "one down," taking revenge, getting even, getting back at others.

VICIOUSNESS: Going for the throat, hitting below the belt, taking pleasure in causing pain in others, intentional cruelty.

PUNITIVENESS: Punishing others for what they did, teaching someone a lesson.

AGGRESSION: Pushiness, intrusiveness, bullying, being rude and abrasive.

SULKING: Passively punishing others with a silence that is hostile and controlling.

MANIPULATION: Controlling others indirectly; a way of getting what you want without having to ask for it in a straightforward way.

SCAPEGOATING: Yelling or screaming at the kids, your partner, or your pets; taking out your anger on targets other than the true source of your anger.

What are your indirect ways of expressing anger?

1. . . . .

. . . .

. . . .

. . . .

2. . . . .

. . . .

. . . .

. . . .

3. . . . .

. . . .

. . . .

. . . .

Blocks to Expressing Anger

Women learn to be "nice," which means—among other things—hiding angry feelings. By adulthood, even verbal expression of anger is curtailed. To protect ourselves from the unbearable idea of expressing our angry feelings, we go the next step and convince ourselves that we are not angry, even when we are. Below are some reasons you might feel you cannot or should not be angry.

YOU FEEL YOU OWE THE OTHER PERSON A DEBT OF GRATITUDE. You are unable to express anger because other person has done so much for you. You might think, *How could I possibly be angry, since . . .*

YOU ARE BEING CONTROLLED BY THE OTHER PERSON. This is a variation on debt of gratitude. You are being imposed on by the other person's helplessness, fragility, or illness.

YOU BELIEVE THAT ANGER IS DESTRUCTIVE OR NEGATIVE. You may be confusing action with feeling.

YOU FEAR BEING CALLED NAMES. For example, you don't want to be called a bitch.

YOU JUDGE YOURSELF FOR YOUR ANGRY FEELINGS. This usually comes back to what you learned about anger as a child. You might think, *If I get angry, I'm bad.*

YOU NEED TO LOOK GOOD. You have an idealized self-image. You want people to see you as easygoing. You don't want to damage your outward appearance.

YOU BELIEVE THAT EXPRESSION OF ANGER IS TRAUMATIC. You have vowed never to get angry because you experienced violence in your family as a child.

YOU FEAR RETALIATION. Perhaps you were beaten down or humiliated for expressing anger in the past, and you want to avoid repeating that experience.

YOU HAVE A SECONDARY AGENDA. You have an investment in a certain outcome, and if you risk anger, you might not get what you want. You may use manipulation to get your way.

YOU DON'T UNDERSTAND ANGER. You may be naive about feelings in general, especially anger. Anger is a feeling.

YOU ARE SCARED OF THE ENERGY RELEASED BY ANGER. You may believe that anger leads to assertiveness, which leads to power, which leads to aloneness.

YOU FEAR YOUR OWN ANGER. You may not trust your anger. You fear you may be violent, punitive, or sadistic if you let your anger out.

Telling yourself that you're not angry or squelching your anger is seldom completely successful, however, and the blocked anger leaks out in indirect or inappropriate ways.

What are your blocks to expressing anger?

1. . . . .

. . . .

. . . .

. . . .

. . . .

2. . . . .

. . . .

. . . .

. . . .

3. . . . .

. . . .

. . . .

. . . .

Gender Roles and Anger

In this section, we'll take a look at your beliefs about gender and power; then we'll consider the childhood socialization that shaped these beliefs.

❧

How would you characterize your relationship: as egalitarian, male-dominant, female-dominant, or mixed?

. . . .

. . . .

. . . .

Who makes the important decisions in your home?

. . . .

. . . .

. . . .

. . . .

Do you see yourself as the queen of your castle (home)? Why or why not?

. . . .

. . . .

. . . .

. . . .

When you ask your partner, husband, or boyfriend to help you with household chores, do you supervise him or her?

. . . .

. . . .

. . . .

. . . .

If the household chores are not done according to your standards, do you redo them?

. . . .

. . . .

. . . .

. . . .

Where do you think you picked up these attitudes?

. . . .

. . . .

. . . .

. . . .

How does your partner respond to you if you supervise him or her in doing household chores?

. . . .

. . . .

. . . .

. . . .

❧

A number of social and biological differences exist between men and women. Growing up, most girls play in small groups and make decisions based on mutual agreement. Girls more often play games that involve taking turns and cooperating, such as jump rope or hopscotch. Girls usually suppress their anger and instead engage in gossip and backstabbing behavior (Tannen 1990).

Differences in socialization have consequences in terms of our values, expectations, and motives. These differences are possible sources of anger and conflict. Women usually place a higher value on intimacy than men do. Women tend to engage in dialogue and express feelings more than men do (Tannen 1990).

Childhood Socialization of Gender Roles

Let's take a look at your childhood experiences of socialization and gender roles.

Think back to your childhood. What did you like about being a girl? What did you dislike?

. . . .

. . . .

. . . .

What type of childhood games did you play? Did these games involve cooperating, taking turns?

. . . .

. . . .

. . . .

What were some things you learned about being a girl from your parents, teachers, and classmates?

. . . .

. . . .

. . . .

Would you raise a daughter (or your own, if you have one) the same way you were raised? If not, what would you do differently?

. . . .

. . . .

. . . .

. . . .

Below is a list of habits or tendencies that can indicate hidden anger. Check those habits that best relate to you.

o procrastination in completing tasks that are imposed on you

o perpetual or habitual lateness

o frequent forgetfulness when asked to do something

o frightening thoughts or violent fantasies

o sarcasm, cynicism, or flippancy in conversation

o overpoliteness, constant cheerfulness, or a grin-and-bear-it attitude

o a liking for sadistic or ironic humor

o frequent sighing

o smiling while hurting

o frequent disturbing or frightening dreams

o overcontrolled, monotone speaking voice

o difficulty in getting to sleep or sleeping through the night

o boredom, apathy, loss of interest in things you are usually enthusiastic about

o slowing down of movements

o having less energy, getting tired more easily than usual

o excessive irritability over little things

o getting drowsy at inappropriate times

o sleeping more than usual (twelve to fourteen hours a day)

o waking up tired rather than rested and refreshed

o clenching jaws, especially while sleeping

o facial tics, spasmodic foot movements, habitual fist clenching, and similar repeated physical acts done unintentionally or unaware

o grinding of the teeth, especially while sleeping

o chronically stiff or sore neck or shoulder muscles

o chronic depression, extended periods of feeling down for no reason

o patting or stroking the back of the head

o physical problems such as stomach ulcers, headaches, or colitis

o high blood pressure

o frequent accidents or illnesses

- anxiety attacks: heart palpitations, nausea, chills, sweats, flushing, panic
- compulsive overeating
- overworking, overexercising
- reckless driving, daredevil behavior
- suicidal thoughts or actions
- self-sabotage, expecting failure
- being hypercritical of people, places, or things
- suddenly refusing eye contact with another person
- laughing when nothing amusing is happening
- fidgeting
- loss of interest in being affectionate with your partner

What are some of the other ways you hide anger from yourself and others?

1. . . . .

. . . .

. . . .

. . . .

2. . . . .

. . . .

. . . .

. . . .

3. . . . .

. . . .

. . . .

. . . .

Lesbians and Homophobia

Lesbians face unique challenges when it comes to socialization and anger. *Homophobia* is the fear, dread, or hatred of homosexuality. Homophobia is an intricate system of stereotypes, myths, and half-truths that serve to enforce traditional sex roles and male dominance.

Internalized homophobia keeps lesbians feeling ashamed and experiencing low self-esteem. Many lesbians choose to be invisible, or closeted, which then makes them unable to know themselves. Homophobia can lead lesbians to hurt themselves and others.

It is sometimes difficult to separate external and internalized homophobia. For example, the gay and lesbian community has justifiable fears that homophobia will be used against them: they fear the loss of their families, jobs, children, homes, and lives. Most lesbians have received messages of homophobia since early childhood.

These exercises are about personal growth and freedom for lesbians.

❧

What are the conventional expectations of female children?

. . . .

. . . .

. . . .

. . . .

Why is it that around puberty, children begin calling each other "queer" or "lesbo"?

. . . .

. . . .

. . . .

. . . .

What are the images of lesbians you saw as a young girl on TV or in books?

. . . .

. . . .

. . . .

. . . .

If the media creates a vision of society, where are you in it?

. . . .

. . . .

. . . .

. . . .

List the myths and stereotypes about lesbians. (*All lesbians like to wear men's clothing; Lesbians hate men; Lesbians don't wear makeup;* and so on.)

. . . .

. . . .

. . . .

. . . .

. . . .

. . . .

. . . .

. . . .

❧

As a result of homophobia and heterosexism, many lesbians experience shame in a variety of ways. Shame leads some lesbians to choose to remain closeted and invisible. Others turn to alcohol and drug abuse to help dull the pain and shame they feel. How has internalized homophobia affected you?

. . . .

. . . .

. . . .

. . . .

. . . .

How has internalized homophobia or heterosexism affected your behavior in relationships?

. . . .

. . . .

. . . .

. . . .

. . . .

. . . .

❖

You are not responsible for changing society's attitudes, but you do have control over your own attitude. Consider how internalized homophobia has affected your life. You can empower yourself and repair your self-esteem by choosing a more positive attitude.

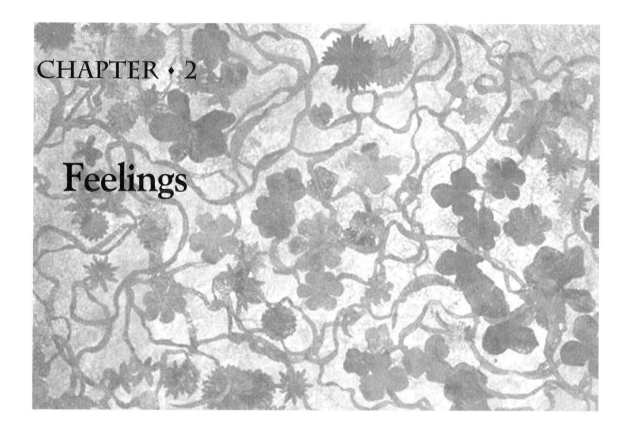

CHAPTER • 2

Feelings

MANY WOMEN in our society have been discouraged from directly expressing or being aware of their feelings and needs. Women have long been the ones who take care of others, who deal with others' hurt, pain, and suffering. Women have been taught to put themselves second. Some women hold on to relationships despite the toll it takes on their own well-being. When we have not learned how to express our feelings and needs, it can be difficult and confusing to even know what we feel and need. We may suddenly find ourselves very angry (or depressed or frustrated) and not know why. Many women learn to "stuff" their feelings at an early age, usually from family experiences. We may have observed our mothers serving as peacemakers and martyrs, going to extremes to avoid conflict. We may have been punished for saying what we felt, or we may have witnessed painful arguments or violent fights between our parents around discussion of feelings. From these experiences we learn to tell ourselves *Don't rock the boat; It's not worth it to express how I really feel;* or *My feelings aren't important.* Instead of acknowledging and expressing our feelings, we ignore them and turn them into secondary feelings of anger or depression.

Defining Your Emotions and Feelings

Understanding and naming your feelings can be difficult and tricky. You may sometimes mask your true feelings, and furthermore, your emotions change all the time. Emotions are reactions you have to things around you, and you use "feeling" words to describe them. Because the events you react to are constantly changing, it's natural that your emotions would change, too. Your emotions can change rapidly, within seconds in some situations.

Because you ride this emotional roller coaster continually, you can get confused about which feeling is attached to which event. Let's take Sandi for an example. Sandi got upset about an argument with her child one morning. She snapped at her daughter, was rude to the coffee shop waiter, and later yelled at her coworker. Sandi believed that the argument with her daughter caused her to become short with everyone else that day.

After talking with Sandi, I learned that she had a very important presentation later in the day and had spent much of the previous night preparing—and worrying, since she had never given a presentation before. Sandi eventually came to admit that she had very little confidence in herself and was fearful of failing miserably. She also came to realize that the argument with her daughter was actually a reaction to her fear and was not what caused her to be moody all day.

Like Sandi, you can learn to understand exactly what you are feeling and what may have precipitated those feelings. First, let's take a look at some of the basic feelings we all have. Do any of the facial expressions on the next two pages look familiar?

HOW DO YOU FEEL?

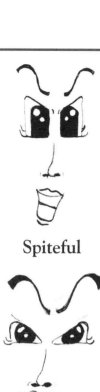

Spiteful

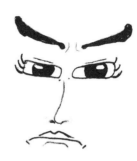

Angry

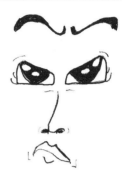

Frustrated

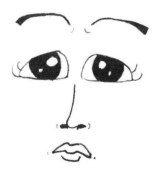

Enraged

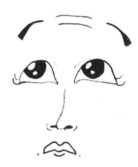

Ashamed

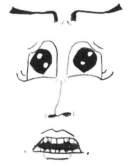

Overwhelmed

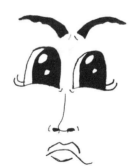

Lonely

Jealous

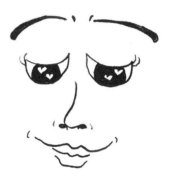

Loving

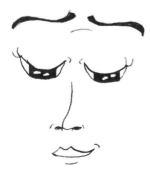

Shy

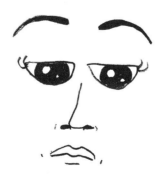

Bored

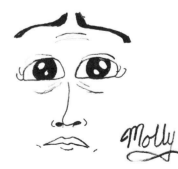

Depressed

HOW DO YOU FEEL?

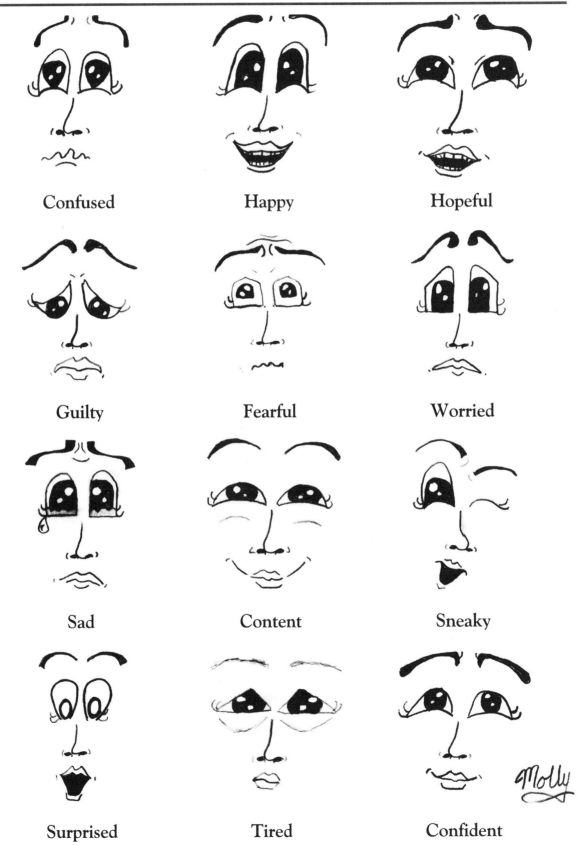

Confused   Happy   Hopeful

Guilty   Fearful   Worried

Sad   Content   Sneaky

Surprised   Tired   Confident

Dealing with Angry Feelings

The process of dealing with angry feelings can be divided into three parts for purposes of discussion, although the living of it is all one piece. The parts are

1. recognizing your feelings,

2. owning your feelings, and

3. responding to your feelings.

RECOGNIZING YOUR FEELINGS

Every woman has her own bodily signals indicating current, on-the-spot feelings. In other words, almost all emotions have some sort of physical reaction to them. Being aware of your physical reaction can help you better understand what emotion you may be feeling. Below are some common physical symptoms for different emotions.

Physical symptom: tight muscles, clenched fists

Emotions: mad, angry, frustrated, spiteful, jealous

Physical symptom: smiling

Emotions: happy, content, pleased, good-humored, excited, proud, confident

Physical symptom: frowning

Emotions: upset, sad, mad, disappointed

Physical symptom: weakness

Emotions: tired, depressed, hopeless

Physical symptom: crying

Emotions: sad, depressed, exhausted, upset, joyful

Physical symptom: lowered head

Emotions: shy, embarrassed, depressed, disgusted, ashamed

Physical symptom: sweating

Emotions: anxious, scared, worried

Physical symptom: speechless

Emotions: shocked, surprised

Physical symptom: blushing

Emotions: embarrassed, shy, guilty, ashamed

Physical symptom: "in a fog"

Emotions: overwhelmed, worried, confused

Physical symptom: butterflies in the stomach

Emotions: nervous, scared, anxious

Think back over the last week or two. What were some of your physical reactions to various emotions? Personalize these symptoms by adding to them or changing them as needed. You may want to ask close family and friends, since they may be aware of particular reactions you cannot see or consciously feel.

Physical symptom: . . . .

Emotions: . . . .

Physical symptom: . . . .

Emotions: . . . .

Physical symptom: . . . .

Emotions: . . . .

When you find yourself depressed or blue and don't know why, think back over the past twenty-four hours and try to figure out who did something to anger you. Forget you are easygoing and imagine yourself to be the toughest, most unreasonable person on earth. Review your day and look for an incident that might have made this person angry.

What was the incident?

. . . .

. . . .

. . . .

Why didn't you get angry?

. . . .

. . . .

. . . .

Chances are you really did get angry, you just didn't know it. Remember what you actually did and said in that situation—try to relive it. Write down any internal anger signals that you can identify from the incident.

. . . .

. . . .

. . . .

. . . .

Pick a recent incident that made you angry. How did you recognize your anger?

. . . .

. . . .

. . . .

. . . .

❧

OWNING YOUR FEELINGS

The anger is yours. The other person may have said or done something that punched your anger button, but the anger is yours, and so are the feelings it triggers. You cannot make someone else responsible for your own feelings. Blaming does not help. Nothing the other person does will help, unless it is in response to something you do.

Accepting anger as your own is easier if you discard the idea that feelings need to be justified. They don't, and frequently cannot be. *Should* and *feel* are two words that do not belong together. It is senseless to say that someone "should feel" some way. Feelings just are there in the same way your skin, muscles, and vital organs are.

RESPONDING TO YOUR FEELINGS

First, foremost, and always: breathe first, and then decide how you want to respond. Anger demands expression; if you have recognized it and owned it, then you will have a choice of when, where, and how you express it. Just saying *That makes me angry* or *I do not like it when . . .* may not be as satisfying as hitting someone, but it has far less serious consequences. There are, however, a few situations in which it is in your best interest to delay expression. For example, if you're angry with your boss, it's better to wait until you are completely calm before you express your anger.

Suppression of Anger and the Volcano Effect

There are many other feelings that contribute to anger. If these primary feelings are not communicated and dealt with, they can boil beneath the surface and eventually cause so much pressure that they erupt in a volcano of secondary emotion: anger.

PRIMARY FEELINGS COMMONLY TURNED INTO ANGER

Here is a list of feelings that can build up and lead to an anger eruption.

HURT: Sadness, feeling choked up, needing to cry.

FEARFUL: Afraid of losing someone or of being hurt, for example.

INSECURE: Feeling unsure of yourself.

IGNORED: Feeling that others aren't paying attention to you.

ISOLATED: Feeling no one is there for you.

INADEQUATE: Thinking you are not good enough.

EMBARRASSED: Feeling ridiculed or put down.

REJECTED: Thinking someone cares more for others than for you.

HUMILIATED: Feeling put down or laughed at.

OUT OF CONTROL: Wanting others to do what you want.

GUILTY: Feeling that you have let others down.

Denying Angry Feelings

Why do women deny their anger? Because as women we were socialized to believe that our anger is not acceptable to others. Many women do not feel worthy of being angry. Take, for instance, a situation where you work. Suppose that your boss grants your coworker time off during an especially busy week, and you know your workload will be much heavier as a result. It is a lot easier just to deny that the situation makes you angry, not make waves, and not have a confrontation. Anger is a feeling we often deny because it is uncomfortable for most of us.

If you grew up in a chaotic home, the turmoil may have been so intense that you learned to deny your anger. Perhaps you felt safer not expressing your anger and hoped it would go away. Chances are you eventually became unaware of its presence. Repressed anger can lead to serious resentment and depression. It causes physical complications that lead to stress-related illnesses.

Denying anger causes problems in relationships when you are not being truthful about your feelings. You may be fearful of alienating people and destroying relationships.

❖

List specific examples of your behavior that show you were angry but denied it.

. . . .

. . . .

. . . .

. . . .

Now list specific examples of your behavior that show you were angry but expressed it.

. . . .

. . . .

. . . .

. . . .

In what situations is it hardest for you to express your anger?

. . . .

. . . .

. . . .

. . . .

❖

This is an area you'll need help with. If you're working with an anger management therapy group, ask for support from the group; if not, ask for help from a trusted friend or family member.

Summing Up Your Feelings

Now that you've had an opportunity to recognize and name some of your feelings, it is important that you identify your most prominent feelings and determine if there are any patterns to your feelings. The best way to achieve this is by tracking your feelings throughout the week. The feelings checklist below is designed to reveal possible triggers or patterns associated with the feelings listed. Be sure to write in at the bottom any additional feelings that directly apply to you.

Once a day during the next week, check off any of these feelings you've had that day. Also note the time of day you had these feelings.

	Mon	Tue	Wed	Thu	Fri	Sat	Sun
challenged							
out of control							
resistant							
shocked							
uncomfortable							
ambivalent							
frustrated							
filled with hate							
hopeless							
pessimistic							
hurt							
ready to fight							
pressured							
pissed off							
bothered							
sad							
worried							
loving							
boiling mad							
angry							
caring							
jealous							
irritated							
vulnerable							

	Mon	Tue	Wed	Thu	Fri	Sat	Sun
defeated							
furious							
resentful							
explosive							
enraged							
anxious							
burned up							
ignored							
disappointed							
annoyed							
insecure							
growth oriented							
aggravated							
depressed							
threatened							
offended							
upset							
fearful							
confused							
put off							
hopeful							
left out							
violent							
optimistic							
cross							
motivated							

At the end of the week, review your checklist. It is important that you not wait any longer than a week, as it may be difficult to remember details of the incidents.

What are the three most checked feelings for the week?

1. . . . .

2. . . . .

3. . . . .

Were there any particular major events that took place near some of the checked emotions?

. . . .

. . . .

. . . .

. . . .

What emotion most commonly followed these events?

. . . .

. . . .

. . . .

. . . .

Do you see any patterns for your emotions? Some examples might be

❧ I usually feel *insecure* after having a conversation with my boss.

❧ I feel *resentful* when I'm talking with my sister.

❧ I feel *aggravated* every time we all sit down for dinner.

❧ . . . .

❧ . . . .

❧ . . . .

❧ . . . .

Now review your list again, but this time note the days when you checked several different feelings. Do you see one particular feeling following another particular feeling? For instance, if you usually feel insecure after having a conversation with your boss, you might notice that after feeling insecure, you tend to get furious when you're talking with your partner. List any sequence of feelings you experienced.

. . . .

. . . .

. . . .

. . . .

. . . .

❧

Look at the feelings checklist. Select a feeling that describes how you feel *right now*. Now take some paper, crayons, paint, glue (whatever art materials you have on hand) and make a picture of how you feel. If you are in a group setting, share this with the group.

Look at the feelings checklist again. Select a feeling that describes how you usually feel on a day-to-day basis. Now take some paper, crayons, paint, glue (whatever art materials you have on hand) and make a picture of how you feel. If you are in a group setting, share this with the group.

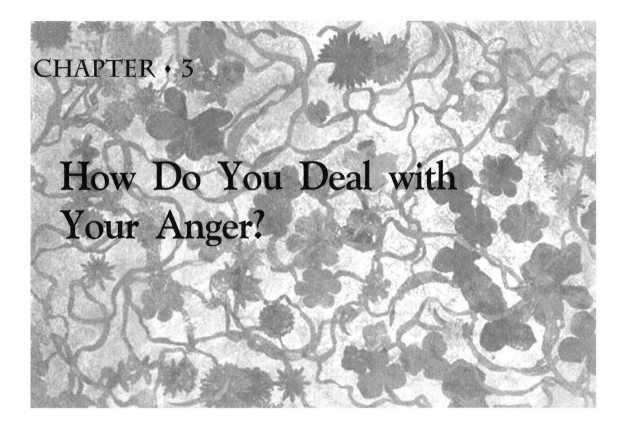

CHAPTER · 3

How Do You Deal with Your Anger?

ANGER IS an emotion that says, *Something is wrong.* It can be expressed to tell others about your personal limits, values, rules, and boundaries. Sandra Thomas defines anger as "a strong, uncomfortable emotional reaction to another person or event that offends our beliefs about the way things should be in a particular situation" (1993, 12). The respectful expression of anger is an important way to educate others about how their behavior affects you. It can result in mutual respect between you and another person.

Not everyone defines anger the same way. Here are different definitions that clients gave.

Anger is a response to pain.

I looked up the word "anger" in the dictionary. The definition I found was "a feeling of extreme displeasure, hostility, indignation, or exasperation toward someone or something; rage; wrath." It also means trouble or pain. To me, anger is pain. Anger is what currently fuels my life. I do not want that. I do not want anger or pain in my life anymore.
   —Wanda

Anger is feeling out of control.

Anger, to me, is like having a hit man inside of me. It is an emotion that takes me over and causes me to explode. I keep my feelings inside because I do not trust anyone with them. I cannot open up these feelings to anyone anymore. When I feel angry, I feel lost,

sad, and mad at everyone because I have so much stored inside of me. I feel like crying, hitting walls, and drinking when anger is present in me.
 —Denise

Anger is a response to hurt and betrayal.

I express it in inappropriate ways in situations that seem unfair to me. I tend to get angry in situations that are beyond my control and I have no power or authority to change.
 —Fran

Anger is a feeling of rage.

Anger is a feeling of heated rage, which is overwhelming and stressful. I find myself angry when I become irritated or harassed by another person.
 —Sheryl

Anger is a response to being ignored.

My boyfriend's mother, when she's upset at me, communicates this by ignoring me rather than telling me what is on her mind. This in turn brings up anger in me.
 —Evelyn

Anger is a response to injustice.

My most recent incident of anger was at work. A patient threw paperwork at me and told me she didn't like the way it was worded. I just felt my blood boiling but maintained my composure. I had to finish with her by having her sign the paperwork, and once she did, I snatched it from her. I made sure I did it just enough for her to feel me but not so much as to jeopardize my job.
 —Erica

How Angry Are You?

Not every woman experiences anger the same way or to the same degree. Some women believe that they don't feel anger, when in fact they are suppressing it. Other women feel a considerable amount of anger and learn to express it constructively. Still others are consumed by anger that hurts them and the people around them. This exercise, developed by Roland Maiuro, will help you determine the role that anger plays in your life.

Read the statements listed below. Rate each one so that it describes your current way of feeling. Circle one answer.

1. When I really lose my temper, I am capable of hitting or slapping someone.

0	1	2	3	4
Extremely unlikely	Unlikely	Possible	Likely	Very likely

2. I get mad enough to hit, throw, or kick things.

0	1	2	3	4
Extremely unlikely	Unlikely	Possible	Likely	Very likely

3. I easily lose my patience with people.

0	1	2	3	4
Extremely unlikely	Unlikely	Possible	Likely	Very likely

4. If someone doesn't ask me to do something in the right way, I will avoid doing it or not do it at all.

0	1	2	3	4
Extremely unlikely	Unlikely	Possible	Likely	Very likely

5. At times I feel I get a raw deal out of life.

0	1	2	3	4
Extremely unlikely	Unlikely	Possible	Likely	Very likely

6. When I get mad, I say threatening or nasty things.

0	1	2	3	4
Extremely unlikely	Unlikely	Possible	Likely	Very likely

To score this exercise, add the numbers circled in each question. If your score is lower than 5, you express your anger constructively. If your score is between 5 and 9, you have a problem expressing your anger constructively. If your score is 10 or higher, you express your anger in an abusive way and could benefit from an anger management program.

Types of Anger

Anger is not a one-size-fits-all emotion. Everyone feels and expresses anger in a personalized way. Anger can be experienced and expressed in three systems: *behavioral* (our actions), *cognitive* (our thoughts and images), and *physiological* (our body's response).

BEHAVIORAL ANGER

Crying, shouting, shoving, and hitting are examples of behavioral anger. Sandra Thomas (1993) discovered during her study of women and anger that women frequently express their anger by crying. June Crawford and her colleagues state that crying is "a signal of the righteousness of women's anger along with the strength of the hurt" (1992, 176). Because women grow up in a society that does not validate women when they express anger, many women cry when they are angry so that their anger might be more acceptable to others.

A woman can express anger by crying and physically acting out, which then leads her to feel guilty and embarrassed. Anne Campbell (1993) suggests women cry when they are angry because they feel that anger or aggression represents a kind of failure on their part.

Sharon explains how she shows anger.

When I am angry, I often show it in physical ways, by hitting or scratching or other physical means. When I argued with my ex-boyfriend, I would scratch his chest. This was my way of releasing the intense anger in me and showing him how angry I was.

You can recognize behavioral anger by noticing facial expression, body posture, the language you use, and how loud you are. Cristy relates her story:

When my partner and I woke up in the morning, we were just lying on the bed, and I jokingly said, "You were pretty cranky last night." I was not prepared for her response back to me. "I was trying to give you space last night because you seemed to need it." In a matter of moments, my emotional response escalated and I was standing up, my hands on my hips, yelling at my partner. I had to walk out because I got so upset. I was angry with myself for not having the ability to just listen to what my partner had to say instead of getting defensive and all worked up.

Define your behavioral anger. List the actions and behaviors you exhibit when you are angry.

1. . . . .

2. . . . .

3. . . . .

COGNITIVE ANGER

Cognitive anger refers to our thoughts and images. Angry thoughts can come very quickly, almost automatically. These thoughts may be accurate, but often they are inaccurate or exaggerated. Saying such things to yourself can increase and prolong your anger.

I had a friend who was unattractive, but extremely witty and fun to hang out with. She also had a big ego that was annoying. She would have temper tantrums whenever she didn't get any attention. So one night she went off on me. I got the brunt of her anger.

She tried to make fun of my style and my looks. She herself was unattractive, so people would avoid making negative comments about her looks. I was pissed that she would even go there with me. So I shut her out as a friend and made fun of her. I nicknamed her the Troll. But the thing was, when I called her that name, I was the one who became angrier.

    —Penny

Cognitive images are the pictures in your mind of how things "should" be. When real life doesn't meet the image, you can become frustrated and angry.

When I am very angry, I remember things that occurred in my past relationship. I then feel underestimated by that person and want to hurt him. I become angry when I see him happy with another, especially when he has destroyed our relationship.

    If I am angry with someone, I tend to think others don't like me and are happy seeing me having problems. These feelings I harbor inside affect my self-esteem, and I think a lot about my failures and unhappy times.

    When I am angry, I feel it is an opportunity to let out all the things I hold inside, things that are sitting there, eating me up. I release all the pain inside at the person who's in front of me at that time.

    —Yvette

Define your cognitive anger. List the thoughts and images you are aware of when you are angry.

1. . . . .

. . . .

. . . .

2. . . . .

. . . .

. . . .

3. . . . .

. . . .

. . . .

PHYSIOLOGICAL ANGER

Anger is not only expressed in your behavior and in your brain, it is also expressed in your body. In fact, sometimes when women are not aware of their anger, it can show physically, like Karen explains:

I feel anger in a physiological way. I was at court last Thursday, and my social worker informed me that my boyfriend, who was also present, could not ask the judge to dismiss the restraining order. He had been told by my other social worker that he would be able to. I felt my heart racing, and my face became hot and red.

The physiological system includes the nerves, respiratory system, muscles, heart, blood vessels, stomach and intestines, and endocrine glands. When you are angry, some physiological cues could be shortness of breath, rapid breathing, flushed face, sweating, a knot in your stomach, or rapid heartbeat. When the physiological response to anger occurs too often or lasts too long, it can be stressful. This stress can result in anxiety attacks, headaches, nausea, depression, or more serious medical problems.

Define your physiological response to anger. List what happens to your body when you are angry.

1. . . . .

2. . . . .

3. . . . .

What does your anger look like? Using a pen and paper, or any art materials you have on hand, make a picture of what your anger looks like. How did you feel making this picture of your anger?

If you're working in a group, create a collage together on a large piece of paper showing what your anger looks like and feels like. How did it feel to make a picture of your anger in a group, compared to making your own picture? What was similar or different?

. . . .

. . . .

. . . .

. . . .

. . . .

. . . .

Anger Triggers

A woman's anger is triggered for a variety of reasons. Thomas's study (1993) revealed three common themes that trigger women's anger: powerlessness, injustice, and the irresponsibility of other people. Other triggers include interpersonal relationships; being treated unfairly; unmet expectations; feeling stressed-out, pressured, disrespected, criticized, tired, threatened, or harassed; someone else's thoughtlessness; and incompetence.

To identify your anger triggers, use the checklist below created by Thomas (1993).

What triggers your anger?

- unfair treatment

- the unfair treatment of someone I care about (family member, friend, coworker, child)

- unmet expectations

- powerlessness

- offense to my morals or values

- stress and pressure

- someone else's thoughtlessness

- someone else's incompetence

- disrespectful treatment

o criticism

o inability to control something or someone

o interference with my goals or plans

o harassment

o delays (traffic, long lines, etc.)

o fatigue

o the irresponsibility of someone I depended on

o property damage or destruction

o threats to my self-esteem

o my own stupidity

o other: . . . .

o . . . .

o . . . .

o . . . .

What situations most likely trigger your anger?

1. . . . .

2. . . . .

3. . . . .

❧

Defining Your Anger Style

The next two exercises will help you identify your personal style of experiencing and expressing anger. Do you tend to stifle your anger and express it indirectly through sulking, manipulation, or punitiveness (anger-in)? Or do you tend to release your anger by yelling or throwing things (anger-out)? What physical sensations accompany your anger? How long does your anger last, and how do you feel afterward?

The next exercise was created by Charles Spielberger.

What do you do when you're mad? For each question, choose among "Not too likely" (one point), "Somewhat likely" (two points), and "Very likely" (three points).

When really angry or annoyed, you:

a. Try to act as though nothing happened.

1	2	3
Not too likely	Somewhat likely	Very likely

b. Keep it to yourself.

1	2	3
Not too likely	Somewhat likely	Very likely

c. Apologize even though you are right.

1	2	3
Not too likely	Somewhat likely	Very likely

d. Get if off your chest.

1	2	3
Not too likely	Somewhat likely	Very likely

e. Talk to a friend or relative.

1	2	3
Not too likely	Somewhat likely	Very likely

f. Blame it on someone else.

1	2	3
Not too likely	Somewhat likely	Very likely

g. Take it out on others.

1	2	3
Not too likely	Somewhat likely	Very likely

h. Get tense or worried.

1	2	3
Not too likely	Somewhat likely	Very likely

i. Get a headache.

1	2	3
Not too likely	Somewhat likely	Very likely

j. Feel weak.

1	2	3
Not too likely	Somewhat likely	Very likely

k. Feel depressed.

1	2	3
Not too likely	Somewhat likely	Very likely

l. Get nervous or shaky.

1	2	3
Not too likely	Somewhat likely	Very likely

Women with high scores on questions a through c are categorized as anger-in. Women with high scores on questions d and e exhibit *anger discussion* (the healthier ways to express anger). Women with high scores on questions f and g are categorized as anger-out. Women with high scores on questions h through l have strong anger symptoms (exhibit signs of unhealthy anger expression).

The next exercise, the Women's Daily Anger Journal, was created by Sandra Thomas (1993).

Make at least ninety photocopies of the anger journal. Make it into a notebook and carry it around with you. It's important to analyze each anger incident as soon as it happens, while it's still fresh in your mind. After you have kept your journal for at least ninety days, look for recurring patterns and themes.

Women's Daily Anger Journal

The Anger Incident

What happened? . . . .

. . . .

. . . .

. . . .

. . . .

First Reaction

When I got angry, I was thinking . . . .

. . . .

. . . .

. . . .

. . . .

Anger Tactics Checklist

My anger was

o suppressed (kept to myself)

o vented outwardly by screaming, yelling, swearing, or making sarcastic remarks

o released by talking it over with a confidant (spouse, friend, etc.)

o released through vigorous exercise or physical activities

o released by throwing or breaking things

o released through a nasty note or memo

o expressed through pouting or sulking

o expressed in an assertive manner to the person who provoked it

Physical Sensations and Reactions

My anger was accompanied by

o crying

o a tight, knotted feeling in the stomach

o headaches

o a stiff neck

o a pounding heart

o clenched fists

o faster breathing

o lumps in the throat

o shakiness

o eating and more eating

o smoking

o drinking

o taking drugs

o other

Anger Intensity

On a scale from 1 to 10, how strong was my anger? . . . .

Anger Duration

I remained angry for . . . . (minutes, hours, all day, longer).

Anger Aftermath

Afterward I felt

o tense, nervous

o guilty, remorseful

o depressed, sad

o mad at myself

o helpless

o embarrassed

o defeated

o ashamed of myself

o proud of myself

A Just Anger

Anger shines through me
Anger shines through me
I am a burning bush.
My rage is a cloud of flame.
My rage is a cloud of flame
In which I walk
Seeking justice
Like a precipice.
How the streets
Of the iron city
Flicker, flicker,
And the dirty air
Fumes.
Anger storms
Between me and things
Transfiguring
Transfiguring.
A good anger acted upon
Is beautiful as lightning
And swift with power.
A good anger swallowed,
A good anger swallowed
Clots the blood
To slime.

—Marge Piercy,
Circles on the Water

Write a poem that describes your anger. Share it with a friend, or, if you are working with a group, share it with the group.

. . . .

. . . .

. . . .

. . . .

. . . .

. . . .

Art Therapy and Anger

My daughter loves to paint and draw. She enjoys putting her artwork on the walls of our house and on the refrigerator door. But all too often, when we become adults, we abandon this important soul task of childhood. When we grow up, we think of art as something to be shown in an art gallery. We no longer create our own art to convey our feelings. We expect to be able to express our anger rationally, but this does not convey the full extent of our angry feelings. Artists have tried to tell us for years that art is not about the expression of talent or the making of pretty things. Art is about the making of life. Art can be about expressing anger in a creative way.

There are many ways you can use art therapy to heal your anger control problems. The essential process of healing with art involves a deep personal change on your part. You can start to heal by opening up your inner voice.

How do art and music heal? In their book *Creative Healing* (1998), Mary Rockwood Lane and Michael Samuels tell us that art heals by changing a woman's physiology and attitude. The body's physiology changes from a state of stress and anger to one of deep relaxation, creativity, and inspiration. Art and music put you in a different brain wave pattern; art and music affect your *autonomic nervous system* (the part of the nervous system that controls the heart rate, among other things), hormonal balance, and brain neurotransmitters.

Art and music affect every cell in the body instantly to create a healing physiology and attitude. Art and music can change your perception of your world. They create hope and positivity, and they help you cope with your anger and stress. Art therapy helps you see how your anger looks—that part of your anger that you are not aware of. It is a safe way to express strong, angry, and sometimes destructive emotions.

During my doctoral internship in Seattle, Washington, I was fortunate to have my sister Celia Van Maarth, who is an art therapist, living nearby. She volunteered her time and expertise by facilitating this art therapy exercise for my anger management group for women. You can do this exercise by yourself or with a group.

First, it is important to clear a space where you can work. Gather some magazines, construction paper, tape or glue, markers, and any other art materials you have on hand, such as feathers, glitter, crayons, paint, and paintbrushes. Getting the art materials together and looking at the materials makes a space to create.

Remind yourself not to judge yourself. This exercise is not about being an artist; it's about using art to explore feeling and emotions. It's about seeing feelings and making them visible to you. It is the process that is important, not the product.

Make a collage about growing up in your family. Using the magazines, cut out words, phrases, or pictures. Let your unconscious make the choices; don't think too much about it. Keep cutting things out until you are finished. Arrange the things you've cut out on a large piece of construction paper.

What does the collage mean to you? What was it like to make it?

. . . .

. . . .

. . . .

. . . .

. . . .

. . . .

Music Therapy and Anger

"Music hath charms to soothe the savage breast."
—William Congreve, *The Mourning Bride*

Music therapy can help you move toward physical, emotional, mental, and spiritual wholeness and help you develop independence, freedom to change, adaptability, balance, and integration. The musical elements of rhythm, melody, and harmony can help you access and then release deep feelings, including anger. Music therapy brings about gradual changes that can subtly but surely optimize the quality of your life.

WHAT DOES MUSIC THERAPY DO?

Music therapy can

❖ facilitate creative expression when you have trouble speaking or expressing yourself;

❖ provide motivation and learning experiences of all kinds;

❖ create the opportunity for positive, successful, and pleasurable social experiences not otherwise available to you; and

❖ help you develop awareness of yourself, others, and your environment, which helps you function better on all levels, enhances your well-being, and fosters independent living.

Music can calm you down when you feel angry or upset, and it can also help energize you and release your angry feelings.

Depending on your style of anger, or what you feel would help you most at the time, choose one of the following. If you tend to experience anger-out, try the first one; if you experience anger-in, try the second one. You can do this alone or in a group setting.

- ❧ Pick a song or CD of calming music that helps you relax, breathe easier, and feel calmer. Take at least fifteen minutes a day to listen to this music.

- ❧ Pick a song or CD that really gets you going. Dance, run, jump around, hit a pillow: get your anger energy out (safely)!

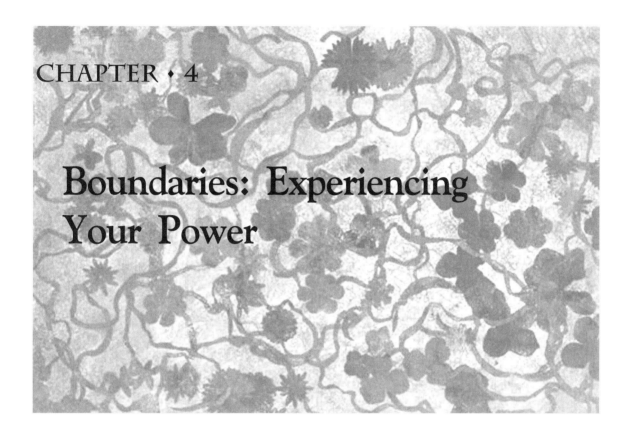

CHAPTER · 4

Boundaries: Experiencing Your Power

THIS CHAPTER, on personal boundaries, will help you come to a deeper understanding of yourself and your relationships.

The following survey, from *Boundaries and Relationships* by Charles L. Whitfield, will help you check out your own personal boundaries and limits.

Survey on Personal Boundaries

For a number of reasons, it may be useful to check out what your boundaries are like now. You may have grown up in a family where healthy boundaries were neither modeled nor taught. You may have been—and may still be—in one or more relationships where you are unclear about boundaries and limits.

1. I can't make up my mind.

| Never | Seldom | Occasionally | Often | Usually |

2. I have difficulty saying no to people.

| Never | Seldom | Occasionally | Often | Usually |

3. I feel as if my happiness depends on other people.

| Never | Seldom | Occasionally | Often | Usually |

4. It's hard for me to look a person in the eyes.

Never   Seldom   Occasionally   Often   Usually

5. I find myself getting involved with people who end up hurting me.

Never   Seldom   Occasionally   Often   Usually

6. I trust others.

Never   Seldom   Occasionally   Often   Usually

7. I would rather attend to others than attend to myself.

Never   Seldom   Occasionally   Often   Usually

8. Others' opinions are more important than mine.

Never   Seldom   Occasionally   Often   Usually

9. People take or use my things without asking me.

Never   Seldom   Occasionally   Often   Usually

10. I have difficulty asking for what I want or what I need.

Never   Seldom   Occasionally   Often   Usually

11. I lend people money and don't seem to get it back on time.

Never   Seldom   Occasionally   Often   Usually

12. Some people I lend money to don't ever pay me back.

Never   Seldom   Occasionally   Often   Usually

13. I feel ashamed.

Never   Seldom   Occasionally   Often   Usually

14. I would rather go along with another person or other people than express what I'd really like to do.

Never   Seldom   Occasionally   Often   Usually

15. I feel bad for being so "different" from other people.

Never   Seldom   Occasionally   Often   Usually

16. I feel anxious, scared, or afraid.

Never   Seldom   Occasionally   Often   Usually

17. I spend my time and energy helping others so much that I neglect my own wants and needs.

Never   Seldom   Occasionally   Often   Usually

18. It's hard for me to know what I believe and what I think.

Never   Seldom   Occasionally   Often   Usually

19. I feel as if my happiness depends on circumstances outside of me.

Never   Seldom   Occasionally   Often   Usually

20. I feel good.

Never   Seldom   Occasionally   Often   Usually

21. I have a hard time knowing what I really feel.

Never   Seldom   Occasionally   Often   Usually

22. I find myself getting involved with people who end up being bad for me.

Never   Seldom   Occasionally   Often   Usually

23. It's hard for me to make decisions.

Never   Seldom   Occasionally   Often   Usually

24. I get angry.

Never   Seldom   Occasionally   Often   Usually

25. I don't get to spend much time alone.

Never   Seldom   Occasionally   Often   Usually

26. I tend to take on the moods of people close to me.

Never   Seldom   Occasionally   Often   Usually

27. I have a hard time keeping a confidence or secret.

Never   Seldom   Occasionally   Often   Usually

28. I am overly sensitive to criticism.

Never   Seldom   Occasionally   Often   Usually

29. I feel hurt.

Never   Seldom   Occasionally   Often   Usually

30. I tend to stay in relationships that are hurting me.

Never   Seldom   Occasionally   Often   Usually

31. I feel an emptiness, as if something is missing in my life.

Never   Seldom   Occasionally   Often   Usually

32. I tend to get caught up "in the middle" of other people's problems.

Never   Seldom   Occasionally   Often   Usually

33. When someone I'm with acts up in public, I tend to feel embarrassed.

Never   Seldom   Occasionally   Often   Usually

34. I feel sad.

Never   Seldom   Occasionally   Often   Usually

35. It's not easy for me to really know in my heart about my relationship with a Higher Power or God.

Never   Seldom   Occasionally   Often   Usually

36. I prefer to rely on what others say about what I should believe and do about religious or spiritual matters.

| Never | Seldom | Occasionally | Often | Usually |

37. I tend to take on or feel what others are feeling.

| Never | Seldom | Occasionally | Often | Usually |

38. I put more into relationships than I get out of them.

| Never | Seldom | Occasionally | Often | Usually |

39. I feel responsible for other people's feelings.

| Never | Seldom | Occasionally | Often | Usually |

40. My friends or acquaintances have a hard time keeping secrets or confidences that I tell them.

| Never | Seldom | Occasionally | Often | Usually |

ASSESSING AND SCORING

In your answers to this survey, many responses of "Usually" and "Often" tend to indicate more boundary problems, distortions, or issues. These may also indicate some confusion over boundaries and limits, often called "blurred" or "fused" boundaries. Women who answered all or mostly "Never" may not be aware of their boundaries. A woman who has healthy boundaries would tend to answer "Seldom" and sometimes "Occasionally."

If you have any questions about any of these areas and dimensions of boundaries and limits, ask your therapist, counselor, therapy group, or other appropriate person.

CONSIDERING YOUR SURVEY ANSWERS

To explore your answers to each of the questions in the survey further, you may wish to discuss them with a therapist. Doing so will allow you to go deeper into your understanding of healthy and unhealthy boundaries and limits in your relationships and your life.

SORTING OUT YOUR BOUNDARIES

It may be helpful now to begin to summarize areas in which you may have some boundary issues or problems. To do so, refer to your answers from the survey. Underline or circle the key words or phrases to which you answered "Usually," "Often," and "Never." While some "Nevers" may not indicate a boundary issue for you, many will. If you are uncertain, ask for feedback from other women.

What Are Boundaries?

Webster's New World Dictionary defines a boundary as "any line or thing marking a limit, a border." In recovery from anger control difficulties, boundaries are a primary issue. Setting a boundary means establishing the lines and limits of our personal territory. Setting a boundary could mean telling a coworker that you won't cover for her when she's late for work. It could mean telling a relative that it's not okay with you that she arrives late to every family gathering and that you will no longer wait until she arrives to sit down to dinner. It could mean telling your partner that you will not allow him to spend time with your children if he continues to make fun of them.

You might be surprised by the idea that you need to set boundaries even if you are not being abused. You can think of it this way: *I'm not trying to keep somebody out of my space, and I'm not trying to keep somebody from abusing me or hitting me. I just think I would be more comfortable if I had some boundaries.*

Try patting your head with one hand and rubbing your tummy with the other hand at the same time. You probably wind up patting with both hands or rubbing with both hands. Unless you concentrate, it's hard to pat with one hand while rubbing with the other. That's a little how relationships are, if patting your head represents watching out for your own boundaries and rubbing your tummy represents respecting other people's boundaries. It's easy to lose concentration, but your goal is to be able to do both things at the same time.

Take a few moments to visualize your own boundary: the lines and limits of your personal territory. What does your boundary look like?

. . . .

. . . .

. . . .

Is it low to the ground, or high up to the ceiling?

. . . .

How thick is the boundary? Is it solid or soft?

. . . .

What are some boundaries you've set in your life?

. . . .

. . . .

. . . .

Can you remember how you felt before and after you set those boundaries?

. . . .

. . . .

. . . .

What are the most difficult kinds of limits for you to set and enforce?

. . . .

. . . .

. . . .

Is someone in your life using you or treating you with disrespect?

. . . .

. . . .

. . . .

Are you angry or complaining? (In other words, is there a boundary you need to set but haven't?)

. . . .

. . . .

. . . .

. . . .

What prevents you from taking care of yourself?

. . . .

. . . .

. . . .

. . . .

What do you think will happen to you if you do set boundaries?

. . . .

. . . .

. . . .

. . . .

What do you think will happen if you don't?

. . . .

. . . .

. . . .

. . . .

How do you feel when you're around people with rigid boundaries (too many rules and regulations)?

. . . .

. . . .

. . . .

How do you feel when you're around people with few or no boundaries?

. . . .

. . . .

. . . .

In the past, what have you been willing to lose for the sake of a relationship?

. . . .

. . . .

. . . .

❧

Creating Healthy Boundaries

Nobody is born with boundaries (Lerner 1985). Our original bond with our caregiver determines how we bond with others. Many women grow into adulthood with damaged, scarred, or nonexistent boundaries. Diseases like chemical dependency and drug abuse or growing up in a domestically violent family affect boundary development. Children growing up in these circumstances may develop an emotional shell no one can get through.

You probably have weak or nonexistent boundaries if, as child, you were emotionally or physically neglected or abandoned. Abuse, humiliation, or shame may have damaged your boundaries. Inappropriate generational roles (such as taking care of a parent when your parent was supposed to be taking care of you) may have confused your boundaries.

One of the goals of recovery from dysfunctional anger is to develop healthy boundaries.

WHAT DOES IT MEAN TO CREATE HEALTHY BOUNDARIES?

Many of us have developed a high tolerance for pain, discomfort, and boundary violation. But how can we tell someone to stop hurting us if we don't know we're hurting? How can we know what we want?

Setting boundaries is not an isolated process. It is intertwined with growing in self-esteem. It means dealing with feelings. It means breaking rules. It means developing spiritually. It means dealing with shame. The more we grow in healing, the better we become at setting boundaries. Boundaries are the key to loving relationships.

A CHECKLIST ON BOUNDARIES IN A RELATIONSHIP

When you give up your boundaries in a relationship, you	When your boundaries are intact in a relationship, you
o are unclear about your preferences	o have clear preferences and act upon them
o do not notice unhappiness, since enduring is your concern	o acknowledge your moods and circumstances, while remaining centered
o do more and more for less and less	o do more when that gets results
o take as truth the most recent opinion you've heard	o trust your own intuition while being open to others' opinions
o live hopefully while wishing and waiting	o live optimistically while cooperatively working on change
o are satisfied if you are coping and surviving	o are only satisfied if you're thriving
o have few hobbies because you have no attention span for self-directed activity	o have excited interest in self-enhancing hobbies and projects
o make exceptions for a person for things you would not tolerate in anyone else; accept alibis	o have a personal standard, albeit flexible, that applies to everyone and asks for accountability
o are manipulated by flattery so that you lose objectivity	o appreciate feedback and can distinguish it from attempts to manipulate
o try to create intimacy with a narcissist	o relate only to partners with whom mutual love is possible

o are so strongly affected by another that obsession results	o are strongly affected by your partner's behavior and take it as information
o will forsake every personal limit to get sex or the promise of it	o integrate sex so that you can enjoy it, but never at the cost of your integrity
o see your partner as causing your excitement	o see your partner as stimulating your excitement
o feel hurt and victimized but not angry	o let yourself feel anger, say "ouch," and embark upon a program of change
o act out of compliance and compromise	o act out of agreement and negotiation
o do favors that you inwardly resist (you cannot say no)	o only do favors you choose to do (you can say no)
o disregard intuition in favor of wishes	o honor intuitions and distinguish them from wishes
o allow your partner to abuse your children and friends	o insist others' boundaries be as safe as your own
o mostly feel afraid and confused	o mostly feel secure and clear
o are enmeshed in a drama that is beyond your control	o are always aware of choices
o are living a life that is not yours and that seems unalterable	o are living a life that mostly approximates what you always wanted for yourself
o commit yourself for as long as the other person needs you to be committed (no bottom line)	o decide how, to what extent, and how long you will be committed
o believe you have no right to secrets	o protect your private matters without having to lie or be surreptitious

Reprinted from *The Therapist*, with permission of CAMFT.

HOW TO FOCUS ON YOURSELF

Writing about your thoughts, experiences, and feelings in a journal is a wonderful way to focus on yourself and begin to explore your boundaries.

Keep a journal. Keep it a private document, never to be read by anyone except you; that way you won't feel the need to censor yourself. This will be a private dialogue with yourself. Write in your journal three times a week, or more often if you feel like it. Here are some questions to help you focus.

Where am I in life now?

What's changing about my life?

What do I desire?

What do I fear?

Whom do I care about?

What hurts?

What feels good?

What am I willing to lose?

Is there someone invasive in my life? What kind of boundary do I need to set with this person?

How do people I admire make their boundaries? What do they say? When do they say it?

Remember: Be gentle with yourself.

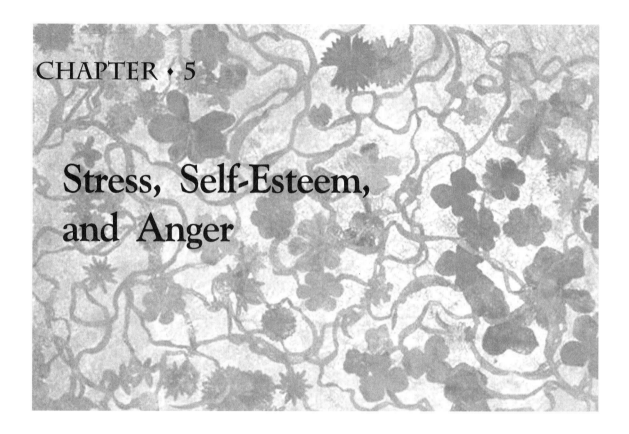

CHAPTER · 5

Stress, Self-Esteem, and Anger

STRESS, SELF-ESTEEM, and anger are all related to each other in complex ways. For example, while it is not clear that stress actually causes anger, it is clear that anger increases with higher levels of stress (Thomas and Donnellan 1993). Self-esteem is also associated with, or goes along with, anger. Researchers have found that women with low self-esteem become angry more easily than women with high self-esteem (Saylor and Denham 1993). Because high stress, low self-esteem, and anger tend to occur together, it is important to understand each concept and to learn how to identify them in your life. This chapter explores each concept and provides some exercises that you may find helpful in understanding how stress, self-esteem, and anger affect your physical and psychological health.

Women and Stress

What is stress? Most people, if asked whether or not they have ever experienced stress, would answer yes. You might, however, have a more difficult time defining exactly what stress is. Although most of us have some general idea about what stress is, many confuse the words *stress* and *stressor*. A *stressor* is some event or situation that puts an excessive physical or psychological demand on a person. *Stress* is an internal bodily response to a stressor. Imagine that you are walking down the street at night and notice that you are being followed by a stranger. Think about how you would feel. Your heart would beat faster, your mouth would become dry, the pupils of your eyes would get bigger, your stomach would tighten, and you would begin to sweat. In this example, the threat of physical harm is the stressor, and the reaction your body has to this threat is stress.

The possibility of physical harm activates a number of chemical reactions in the brain and body that are intended to help you deal with the situation—for example, by running away or fighting back. It is these chemical reactions that cause, among other things, *arousal* (your increased heart rate and blood pressure). Not all stressors are as obvious as the threat of physical harm, but they all activate the same bodily responses.

There are three general categories of stressors:

❧ *Psychological stressors,* such as threats of physical harm, attacks on a person's belief system that cause guilt, and assaults on self-esteem. All of these are situations in which another person attempts to harm you in some way.

❧ *Social stressors,* such as money pressures, war, overcrowding, excessive noise levels, relationship problems, death of a loved one, or other major life changes.

❧ *Biological stressors,* such as physical trauma, diseases and infections, long-term fatigue, and poor nutrition.

Stressors can also be categorized as *normative* or *catastrophic.* Normative stressors are ordinary challenges, like being the parent of a teenager or having the flu. People are usually psychologically prepared for normative stress. When normative stressors are interpersonal, there is usually some kind of fairly comfortable connection between the people involved.

Catastrophic stressors are extraordinary difficulties, like a car accident or the death of a loved one. They create more boundary confusion than normative stressors do. When you're under catastrophic stress, you don't know when the stress is going to end. You are carried from one emotional extreme to another. You may feel isolated. People are generally not psychologically prepared for catastrophic stress.

It seems that just being alive means that we are constantly exposed to a variety of stressors: money problems, looking for a job, getting married, breaking up a relationship, time pressures, meeting deadlines, moving, getting older, and even getting the laundry done. In other words, stress can be caused by a major life event such as the death of a loved one, but stress can also be caused by the buildup of daily hassles. We have all had those days when everything seems to go wrong.

Now that you have a better idea of what stress is, take a few minutes to think about the sources of stress in your life. Use the spaces below to write down the different categories of stressors in your life. Think about whether the stress is *acute* (lasts only a short period of time) or *chronic* (goes on for a long time).

Psychological stressors:

. . . .

. . . .

. . . .

Social stressors:

. . . .

. . . .

. . . .

Biological stressors:

. . . .

. . . .

. . . .

❧

Now that you have had some practice in identifying your sources of stress, you are ready to make your first measurement of your stress level. The Holmes-Rahe scale assigns point values to major life events that cause stress. As you learn to better cope with stress, you can use the scale to measure changes in the amount of stress in your life.

THE HOLMES-RAHE SCALE

Read each of the events listed below, and check the box next to any event which has occurred in your life in the last two years. There are no right or wrong answers. The aim is just to identify which of these events you have experienced lately.

Life Events	Life Crisis Units	Life Events	Life Crisis Units
o Death of spouse	100	o Son or daughter leaving home	29
o Divorce	73	o Trouble with in-laws	29
o Marital separation	65	o Outstanding personal achievement	28
o Jail term	63	o Wife begins or stops work	26
o Death of close family member	63	o Begin or end school	26
o Personal injury or illness	53	o Change in living conditions	25
o Marriage	50	o Revision in personal habits	24
o Fired at work	47	o Trouble with boss	23
o Marital reconciliation	45	o Change in schools	20
o Retirement	45	o Change in residence	20
o Change in health of a family member	44	o Change in work hours or conditions	20
o Pregnancy	40	o Change in recreation	19
o Sex difficulties	39	o Change in church activities	19
o Gain of new family member	39	o Change in social activities	18
o Business readjustment	39	o Mortgage or loan less than $30,000	17
o Change in financial state	38	o Change in sleeping habits	16
o Death of close friend	37	o Change in number of family get-togethers	15
o Change to different line of work	36	o Change in eating habits	15
o Change in number of arguments with spouse	35	o Vacation	13
o Mortgage over $100,000	31	o Christmas alone	12
o Foreclosure of mortgage or loan	30	o Minor violations of the law	11
o Change in responsibilities at work	29		

Your score is: . . . .

Holmes & Rahe (1967). Holmes-Rahe life changes scale. *Journal of Psychosomatic Research*, Vol. 11, pp. 213–218.

According to Holmes and Rahe's statistical prediction model, a score of 150 or less means a relatively low (about 30 percent) probability of stress-related illness (including heart attack, cancer, stroke, etc.). A score of 151 to 299 implies a 50 percent probability and a score of 300 or above implies an 80 percent probability of experiencing a health change—usually a negative change.

The more major life changes you've encountered, the greater your risk of having problems related to stress. If you have a high score, consider the following suggestions:

♣ Become familiar with the life events listed in the scale so you will recognize them as stressors when they happen.

♣ Think about how each life event affects you and how you might best adjust to it.

♣ Take your time in arriving at decisions. Don't be rushed by the event.

♣ If possible, anticipate life changes and plan in advance how you will deal with the extra stress they bring.

♣ Turn the event into a time for positive growth. Look at it as a learning opportunity.

♣ Practice a relaxation activity of your choice.

STRESS AND HEALTH

Why is it important to identify and monitor your stressors and your stress level? Long-term stress—stress that goes on day after day or week after week—will undermine all aspects of your life. While most people can handle short-term stress quite well, chronic stress can result in many psychological and physical health problems.

Stressors cause the brain and body to release a number of different chemicals, including *cortisol* and *adrenaline*, the so-called "stress hormones." Long-term activation of the stress hormones creates an imbalance between body organ systems and leads to many negative health consequences. For example, chronic stress can make you more susceptible to stomach ulcers, stroke, and heart disease. Chronic stress is also known to interfere with the function of your immune system, which fights infections and disease. Because it suppresses immune function, chronic stress has been related to an increased risk of developing a number of infections such as colds and flu. It has also been linked to an increased risk of getting cancer and to the progression of cancer and AIDS. Importantly, chronic stress has been associated with a number of psychological disorders, including anxiety, depression, and post-traumatic stress disorder. Chronic stress can literally damage your brain. One part of your brain that is especially sensitive to the effects of stress is the *hippocampus*. The hippocampus is a brain structure that is very important in new learning and memory. Therefore, chronic stress can disrupt your ability to learn new information.

As you can see, stress is not only related to anger, it is also related to a large number of psychological and physical health problems. Identifying and monitoring your sources of stress is the first step in managing stress and in reducing and preventing stress-related health problems.

DAILY STRESSORS

It is important to pay attention to minor stressors. Researchers have found that daily hassles and problems are an important source of stress and can lead to many of the same health problems that are associated with major stressors (Folkman and Lazarus 1980). Daily hassles and problems could include such things as working with an overly demanding boss, missing a plane flight after a long day of meetings, or juggling the needs of children, home, and work.

❧

What are your daily hassles?

Work:

. . . .

. . . .

. . . .

Home:

. . . .

. . . .

. . . .

Family:

. . . .

. . . .

. . . .

❧

STRESS MANAGEMENT

Managing stress is an important part of learning to cope with anger productively. Stress management is a key to good problem solving. The more you understand your stress, the better you will be able to control it. The more specific you can be in defining your stressors, the more successful you can be at coping with them. In general, stressors that you don't expect (or that you deny will happen) are more likely to cause problems than stressors you expect.

The first step to stress management is identifying the stressful events in your life. The exercise below asks you to sit down at the end of each day and check off the stressful events you experienced that day and the physical symptoms that accompanied them. Look for patterns of times that are more stressful, and you will probably find yourself thinking of other stressors as you do the assignment.

Daily Stressors	MON	TUE	WED	THU	FRI	SAT	SUN
example Stressor: bills arriving in the mail Body clue: shoulders tense		5 P.M.		5 P.M.	5 P.M.		
Stressor: Body clue:							
Stressor: Body clue:							
Stressor: Body clue:							
Stressor: Body clue:							
Stressor: Body clue:							

Which parts of your body are commonly most tense?

. . . .

. . . .

Which of your stressors occur most frequently?

. . . .

. . . .

Most of us live with stress quite successfully. Stress only becomes a problem if you aren't taking good care of yourself and you have an unexpected event. Boundary setting is an important aspect of self-care. Exercise, relaxation, and adequate sleep are other kinds of self-care. By carefully identifying your stressors and the days when your stress is likely to be high, you can plan for better self-care as a way to minimize your stress. You cannot truly prepare for the unexpected. Things will happen over which you have no control. But you can prepare yourself to solve problems creatively when the unexpected happens by carefully identifying your stressors and having a good self-care plan you follow faithfully.

List your self-care activities. Check off the days that you do each activity.

Self-Care Activity	Mon	Tue	Wed	Thu	Fri	Sat	Sun

Self-Esteem and Anger

"No one can make you feel inferior without your consent."
—Eleanor Roosevelt

If you have high self-esteem, you will seldom consent to feeling unnecessarily angry or bad about yourself. Why? Self-esteem is the degree to which you value yourself as a woman, as a human being. The lower your self-esteem, the more likely you are to easily get angry. In addition, women with low self-esteem handle their anger more inappropriately by holding it in or lashing out at others. Unfortunately, these anger tactics get you nowhere fast. The powerful socializing force of sexist gender roles makes women more prone to low self-esteem problems.

1. Perhaps you did not have a childhood that built a strong sense of self-worth. As a young girl, you may not have been given the positive messages needed to create healthy self-esteem. Choose an old photograph of yourself as a child. Place it in a frame and put it on your nightstand. Each night before you go to bed, look at your picture and say something positive to the little girl in the picture:

   You are a survivor.

   I love you.

   You are amazing.

   You are such a smart little girl.

   List your own positive statements here.

   . . . .

   . . . .

   . . . .

   . . . .

2. You are a survivor. List some of the courageous things you did in order to survive your childhood.

   . . . .

   . . . .

   . . . .

   . . . .

3. Set some goals for the soul. List three goals you would like to accomplish in the coming year.

1. . . . .

    . . . .

2. . . . .

    . . . .

3. . . . .

    . . . .

4. Expand your sources of self-esteem. Ask five people you are close to (family or friends) one thing they like about you. Write their responses on a piece of paper, stick it on your mirror, and read it out loud to yourself every morning. If you are not comfortable looking at yourself in the mirror, put the paper on the door and read it to yourself before you go out in the morning.

5. Helen Keller wrote, "Life is either a daring adventure, or nothing." Become a risk taker. Do something you have always wanted to do, but were afraid to.

The one risk I will take this month is

. . . .

. . . .

. . . .

. . . .

. . . .

. . . .

. . . .

❧

"I am me. In all of the world there is no one else exactly like me. There are persons who have some parts like me, but no one adds up exactly like me. Therefore, everything that comes out of me is authentically mine because I alone chose it."
—Virginia Satir

How to Learn Deep Relaxation

The ability to relax deeply and quickly is an extremely useful coping response for dealing with stress, anxiety, or anger. The following exercise, adapted from material by Deffenbacher and colleagues (1987), should allow you to learn this important skill within a week or two. Once mastered, the relaxation response can be used to cope with stress or tension as soon as you feel it beginning to occur. Also, you should experience less stress in your life overall if you practice deep relaxation every day.

Practice the relaxation exercise at least twice a day until you get the hang of it. At first, you will need about thirty minutes of practice. Later, as your skill improves, you will need less and less time to produce the same result.

You may want to have someone read the relaxation instructions aloud to you, or you may want to make a recording, either in your own voice or someone else's.

Practice in a comfortable chair, sofa, or bed, and in a quiet atmosphere. Get as comfortable as possible. Tight clothing should be loosened, and your legs should not be crossed. Take a deep breath, let it out slowly, and prepare to be relaxed as soon as possible. If music helps you to relax, you can play some music while you practice. Finally, it is important to stay awake so that you can compare your feelings of relaxation to your feelings of stress.

1. **Breathe deeply.** This is the key to relaxing quickly and deeply. Breathe slowly, using your abdominal muscles to pull in air all the way down. When you exhale, imagine that you're blowing out stress and tension. Deep breathing can be used anywhere, anytime. If you take too many deep breaths too rapidly, you may become dizzy or light-headed. Breathe slowly, and relax.

2. **Raise your arms and extend them out in front of you.** Now make a fist with both hands as hard as you can. Notice the uncomfortable tension in your hands and fingers. Hold the tension for five seconds, then let the tension out halfway and hold for an additional five seconds. Notice the decrease in tension, but also concentrate on the tension that is still present. Now release the tension completely. Focus on the difference between tensions you felt and the relaxation you now feel. Concentrate on relaxing your hands for ten to fifteen seconds. Breathe deeply.

3. **Tense your upper arms by making a muscle for five seconds.** Focus on the feeling of tension. Then let the tension out halfway for an additional five seconds. Again, focus on the tension that is still present. Now relax your upper arms completely for ten to fifteen seconds and focus carefully on developing relaxation. Let your arms rest limply at your sides. Breathe deeply.

4. **Wrinkle your forehead and scalp as hard as possible.** Hold the tension for five seconds, then release halfway for another five seconds, then relax your scalp and forehead completely. Focus on the developing feeling of relaxation, and contrast it with the tension that existed earlier. Concentrate on relaxing all of the muscles of your body. Breathe deeply.

5. **Clench your teeth, and notice the tension in the muscles of your jaws and mouth.** After five seconds, let the tension out halfway for five seconds, and then relax completely. Let your mouth relax completely with your lips slightly parted, and concentrate on totally relaxing these muscles for ten to fifteen seconds. Breathe deeply.

6. **While keeping the muscles of your chest, arms, and legs relaxed, tense your neck muscles by bringing your head forward until your chin touches your chest.** Hold for five seconds, release the tension halfway for another five seconds, and then relax your neck completely. Allow your head to hang comfortably while you focus on the relaxation developing in your neck muscles. Breathe deeply.

7. **Press the palms of your hands together and push so as to tense your chest and shoulder muscles.** Hold the tension for five seconds, then let the tension out halfway for an additional five seconds. Now relax the muscles completely and concentrate on the relaxation until they are completely loose and relaxed. Concentrate also on the muscle groups (neck, face, forehead and scalp, arms and hands) that have been previously relaxed. Breathe deeply.

8. **Tense your abdominal muscles as hard as possible for five seconds, and concentrate on the tension.** Then let the tension out halfway for an additional five seconds before relaxing your stomach muscles completely. Focus on the spreading relaxation until your stomach muscles are completely relaxed. Breathe deeply.

9. **Extend your legs and raise them approximately six inches above the floor to tense your thigh muscles.** Hold the tension for five seconds, let it out halfway for an additional five seconds, and then relax your thighs completely. Concentrate on totally relaxing your feet, calves, and thighs for about thirty seconds. Breathe deeply.

10. **Point your toes downward so that your feet and calves are tensed.** Hold the tension hard for five seconds, let it out halfway for an additional five seconds, and then relax your feet and calves completely for ten to fifteen seconds. Breathe deeply.

11. **Focus on your whole body and its total relaxation.** You're feeling very warm and peaceful. Continue to breathe slowly and deeply, with very little effort. Begin to bring yourself back into the world around you. You are awake and you are relaxed.

Practice relaxation each day and check it off.

Relaxation	Mon	Tue	Wed	Thu	Fri	Sat	Sun
Week of:							
Week of:							
Week of:							
Week of:							
Week of:							

Which parts of your body were hardest to relax?

. . . .

. . . .

. . . .

. . . .

. . . .

. . . .

. . . .

❧

Self-Esteem and Self-Care

Self-care and self-esteem are tied together. If you don't take care of yourself, you will find your self-esteem will begin to lessen. If you interfere with other people as they try to take care of themselves, you will find both your self-esteem and theirs will begin to drop.

High self-esteem is an accurate appraisal of your strengths and weaknesses. It doesn't mean you feel good and happy all the time. It means you understand both your strengths and weaknesses and are able to make adjustments in your life. If, for example, you have good self-esteem and your workday goes poorly, you will find yourself able to weather the storm better. On the other hand, if your self-esteem is poor, you may find yourself angry, frustrated, tired, depressed, attacking loved ones, drinking excessively, spending money unwisely, or making other decisions that cause problems in your life.

You can build your self-esteem by taking responsibility and being successful. For example, if you take responsibility for your relationships and give them your best effort, your self-esteem will improve. If you take responsibility for your feelings and your life begins to change, your self-esteem will improve.

On the other hand, if you believe that someone else is responsible for your success on the job, and it goes well, your self-esteem may not improve. If you decide other people are responsible for how a relationship goes, your self-esteem will not improve, even if the relationship gets better. If you decide other people cause your feelings, your self-esteem will not improve.

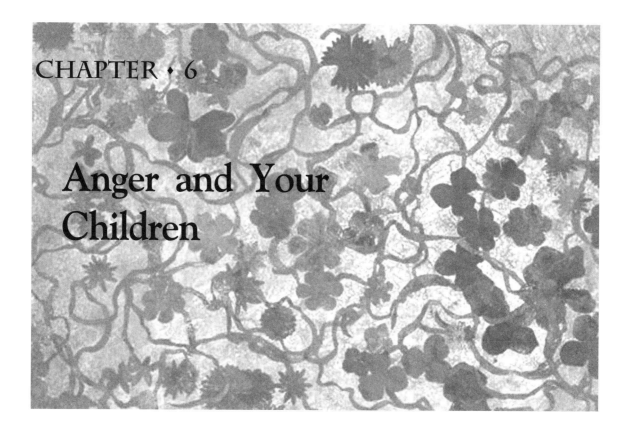

CHAPTER ◆ 6

Anger and Your Children

IF YOU ask any woman, chances are she will tell you that her children are the best things that ever happened in her life. Just don't ask her when her sweet little four-year-old daughter is making a scene at the store or her star thirteen-year-old son gets caught skipping school. If you look over your own list of triggers, your children are very likely near the top. And it's no wonder, when you consider the following factors identified by Thomas and Jefferson (1996, 273):

❖ Women with young children experience high levels of stress, whether they're homemakers or employed outside the home.

❖ Mothers with children under five who don't have a supportive partner are more apt to become clinically depressed than any other group of adults.

❖ Mothers experience higher levels of role overload and conflict than childless women, whether or not those mothers work outside the home.

❖ Women's risk of depression and demoralization is higher if they are mothers of young children. This risk increases with the number of children living at home.

❖ Women retain primary responsibility for childcare (twenty-eight hours per week versus hubby's nine hours per week) even when they work outside the home.

❖ Women are twice as likely as men to experience daily conflict with children.

Start with Yourself

It's no breaking news that most women are so busy taking care of others that they lose sight of themselves. Before a plane takes off, the flight attendant gives one of those rehearsed, informative speeches that, unless you've never flown before, you probably ignore. One of the most important instructions is to be sure to put a mask on yourself before putting it on your children. A lot of research went into that statement; experts found that it is highly possible that a mother would pass out before securing help for her child if she didn't put her own mask on first. In other words, you can't help someone else if you don't help yourself first!

The best way of helping yourself is by learning about your anger. I congratulate you for embarking on that path when you started this workbook. Now, let's take a closer look at your relationship to your children and how your anger affects them.

Comparing Yourself to Your Child

Think it doesn't happen? Ever told yourself that you would never do it? Did you skip this one on your list of triggers? It may be happening without your awareness. If you often hear yourself telling your kids, "I didn't have all the things you do when I was a kid. You have no idea how good you have it," you are probably holding on to some resentment. You may want the best for your child—better than what you had—but somehow you've come to resent it.

My client Frances told me of an incident where she had "lost it." Her ninth-grade daughter kept deliberately missing the bus so she had to be driven to school. Her daughter would even go as far as throwing fits in the morning to arouse an argument that would lead to both of them being late—and resulted in Frances taking her to school. I let Frances continue talking about the latest scene, and eventually the real issue seeped out. "She said that she would look like a geek if she rode the bus. I never got a ride to school when I was her age. If I missed the bus, I had to walk to school and deal with the consequences of being late. Kids today just expect so much—they want to be catered to and are so spoiled."

The conversation continued as Frances reminisced about her own childhood and all the ways it differed from her daughter's. Frances began to display what author Julie Ann Barnhill (2001) refers to as "hidden anger." This anger may be so deep that you simply don't see it. And admitting to this anger is even harder, as it goes against everything we are told a mother is supposed to be. Here are a few examples of ways your child might trigger hidden anger:

* Your child reminds you of someone you intensely dislike or had bad conflicts with in your own childhood.

* Your child is too much like you and has qualities you don't like in yourself.

* Your child is too shy, too lazy about schoolwork, or too unlike other family members and does not conform to your beliefs about the way children should be.

* Your child has become a scapegoat for marital emotions or other stresses within the family system.

* Childcare itself is honestly distasteful to you. You feel resentful and trapped by the responsibilities of parenthood.

List some things that your child has that you didn't.

. . . .

. . . .

. . . .

. . . .

Can you think of any ongoing conflicts with your child that may connect to any of the items you just listed? (Be sure to add these to the anger triggers you listed in chapter 3.)

. . . .

. . . .

. . . .

. . . .

What are some of the things you purposefully provide for your child because you didn't have them yourself?

. . . .

. . . .

. . . .

. . . .

Can you think of a recent incident when you felt some resentment about your child having any of the above-listed items?

. . . .

. . . .

. . . .

. . . .

What issues does your child face that you did not?

. . . .

. . . .

. . . .

. . . .

Is there anyone (from your past or present) whom you dislike and whom your child reminds you of? What are some of the things your child does that remind you of this person? (Add these to your list of anger triggers.)

. . . .

. . . .

. . . .

. . . .

Is there anything you dislike about yourself that you see reflected in your child? (Add these to your list of anger triggers.)

. . . .

. . . .

. . . .

. . . .

What other resentments might you be holding about being a parent? (Add these to your list of anger triggers.)

. . . .

. . . .

. . . .

. . . .

The Drama Game

It is the nature of children to spill things, mess up, and test limits. It's all part of growing up. In fact, in doing so, the child is reaching out to learn. I'm not referring to the type of learning children do in school, but the type of learning that is innate and necessary for life. If you lash out with excessive anger at every little learning incident, you are creating unnecessary drama.

Quite possibly, you are using drama to react to your child's drama. For instance, your child starts crying at a store because you won't buy him the toy he wanted. You are embarrassed by his emotional display and the attention it has drawn. You start out by talking through your teeth in a low voice: "Shut up, you're causing a scene." He calls your drama and raises you one by crying louder and hitting the side of the cart. You double-or-nothing his drama by raising your voice and yelling, "Spoiled brat! Stop crying, or I'll give you something to really cry about!" Maybe you even crown yourself Drama Queen by slapping him.

There are several ways of dealing with this situation, but playing the drama game is not the best. My client Elaine recently encountered a similar situation. Elaine was in a store with her daughter, Ashley. They were in one of those grand stores where a department store and a grocery store are combined. They had spent a lot of time picking out new coats for Elaine, her husband, and Ashley. Ashley was so excited because she was getting a matching hat, scarf, gloves, and purse. But that was hours ago. They were nearing the end of the grocery section when Ashley became restless and irritable. She began screaming, demanded candy, and created a scene. Elaine explained how she handled the situation:

> *I was so surprised at my reaction. It was like I was programmed to make the next move. I didn't say anything, I just took the cart over to the manager, smiled, and said, "I'm so sorry, but my daughter is no longer able to remain in the store and therefore I have to leave. Would you please see that all this is returned to the shelves? I truly apologize." Ashley's eyes grew so big, and she went speechless. I don't know if she was shocked because I didn't do my usual screaming and yelling, or if she was just surprised that we spent all that time shopping and I was willing to just walk away. On the way out, all she could manage to mumble was, "But my coat, and my hat, and my purse . . ." My lack of response was screaming louder than my voice could have. She was sniffling in the backseat, "But what about daddy's coat?" Oh, don't get me wrong—I was so angry, just as angry as I always get when I lose it. But this time I decided to not buy into her drama. I felt some release from the anger as I realized we both had made some progress that day.*

Think of a recent drama where you reacted strongly to your child's actions. What did your child do?

. . . .

. . . .

. . . .

. . . .

What did you do? What did you say to your child?

. . . .

. . . .

. . . .

. . . .

In retrospect, do you see where you might have taken your child's challenge by continuing the drama game? In other words, did you overreact to your child's actions? Step back from the situation and examine what you could have done differently.

. . . .

. . . .

. . . .

. . . .

. . . .

❖

Balancing the Supermom Syndrome

If you are beginning to think that the only reason your children were put on this earth is to test your patience, you're taking it way too personally. Think back to when you were in that idealist state—you know, before your child was born. Your mind probably raced with ideas about the kind of mother you wanted to be and the kind of mother you didn't want to be. You probably formed hopes and dreams about raising your child "right." But that was then, and this is now. Maybe those ideals are just too high to realistically attain. Maybe you found those ideas were actually society's definition of Supermom and not yours. Maybe you just got tired. More than likely, you just came to realize that you are only human. Those dreams are still there; they were just shoved to the back when reality set in.

To understand your anger toward your children, it's good to shine a light on why you are really blowing up. Are you reacting to your children's actions by taking them personally? When your child refuses to pick up her toys, is she really doing it just to piss you off? It's possible that she's just flexing some muscle to see if she really has to follow the rules and if there are consequences for not following those rules.

Staying focused on your beliefs about your job as a mother is essential when working with your anger. I ask all the mothers I work with what roles they identify as being most important for them as mothers. The top five responses I receive are

❧   teacher,

❧   protector,

❧   provider or nurturer,

❧   role model, and

❧   friend or confidant.

❧

What do you believe your role or roles as a mother should be?

. . . .

. . . .

. . . .

. . . .

Reexamine the roles you've just listed and ask yourself if these are society's expectations or your own. Which of those expectations are realistic?

. . . .

. . . .

. . . .

. . . .

For the most part, do you stay focused on these roles when you are angry? Why or why not?

. . . .

. . . .

. . . .

. . . .

If you do stay focused on these beliefs, do you ever feel like you try too hard, setting yourself up for failure with unrealistic expectations?

. . . .

. . . .

. . . .

. . . .

❧

MOM THE TEACHER

A mother knows the right thing to do, when it needs to be done, and does it quickly and efficiently.
—Barbara

Talk about setting goals that will always be out of reach! Barbara's expectations for herself are simply impossible. She may try her best to do and say the right thing, but she's still human. Maybe as a child, you thought your teacher knew everything. But at some point during your life, the curtain was pulled, and the truth about the wizard was revealed.

We all would agree that schoolteachers are very important in our children's lives. You know they're not perfect, but you hope for an honest effort from them. In the movie *Mr. Holland's Opus*, Mr. Holland goes into the field of teaching unwillingly. He teaches straight from a textbook and gets angry when his students don't respond. He is frustrated, and his students are bored and failing. One day, in his frustration, he changes his approach to teaching by connecting to his students in way they can understand. This ignites his students' curiosity, and soon they become engaged. Not only are the kids enjoying the class, but Mr. Holland actually finds himself enjoying teaching.

At first, Mr. Holland hated teaching and acted with anger toward his students. When he finally found a way to connect with them, he realized he could make a difference, and it was possible for them to listen and learn. Many new moms hold a lot of resentment toward their children and lash out with anger. As a mother, you are presented every day with the opportunity to find new approaches and make a difference. Isn't it at least worth a try?

If you place yourself in the same position as a teacher, you may find it easier to deal with your child in ways other than anger. Below is a list of qualities that women claim they want from their children's schoolteachers and some thoughts about how each quality could apply to the mother-child relationship.

BEING PATIENT. This is a very difficult task for women dealing with anger issues. When your child does something that makes you feel angry or upset, you may have to reiterate or change your approach many times before finding the appropriate way to handle this situation. How does a teacher quiet down a room full of screaming kids? By remaining calm, not taking it personally, and trying different approaches until something works.

USING CREATIVITY TO REACH A STUDENT WHO ISN'T GETTING IT. Remember Elaine and her daughter, Ashley? Yelling, rationalizing, and angry outbursts were no longer working. When Elaine used a different approach, she was finally able to put it in a perspective that Ashley could understand.

ENCOURAGING AND EMPOWERING. Parents and sports: what a wicked combination! When a child loses the winning point, don't take it personally, and don't direct anger toward her. Encourage her to keep trying. Empower her by letting her know how proud you are of her for trying, then celebrating her effort.

TEACHING CHILDREN HOW TO THINK, NOT WHAT TO THINK. Debbie's sixteen-year-old daughter May was doing a report and presentation for her history class. May chose the subject of the Inquisition, which is briefly, if ever, covered in school. In both her report and her presentation, she challenged their textbook and called attention to religion's role in the Inquisition. This caused a lot of disruption in the class and the school. It was particularly hard for Debbie, who felt her daughter was "basically trashing our family religion." Debbie eventually came to realize that May had spent many hours researching the topic and took in a lot of considerations to form her opinion. That's what learning is truly about.

We can't expect our children's schoolteachers to teach them everything about life, and we probably wouldn't want them to. Their role is to teach academic lessons, not social, moral, and ethical lessons. If that happens, it's a surprising bonus. As a parent, you are responsible for teaching your child about morals and ethics. If you use your anger to teach these lessons, you are still teaching your children, but not necessarily the lessons you want them to learn.

❧

Think of your favorite teacher in school. Describe this teacher and his or her attributes.

. . . .

. . . .

. . . .

. . . .

. . . .

What are your expectations for a schoolteacher who teaches your child?

. . . .

. . . .

. . . .

Do you extend the same approach to your child? Why or why not?

. . . .

. . . .

. . . .

Think of a recent incident with your child when you reacted with anger. What lesson might you have had the opportunity to teach your child if your anger hadn't gotten in the way?

. . . .

. . . .

. . . .

. . . .

❧

MOM THE PROTECTOR

A mother protects her children from getting hurt or getting in trouble.
　　—Lori

Another impossible task, but worth every ounce of effort you put into it. If you want to protect your children, you have to teach them. Providing your children with the skills to protect themselves will help ease some of your worry.

Lori has dealt with being a "protector" for some time now. She initially came to me after she had used a belt on her children. Lori has two little girls who really enjoy riding their bikes. However, the older one always asked the younger one to ride double on the bike with her. Lori had told them numerous times that it is not safe and they were never to ride that way again. As you can imagine, that didn't stop them. Here is what happened when Lori saw them riding double again.

> *I snapped, as usual. I was just so sick and tired of telling them over and over again. They never listen to me. Plus, I had just found out that their room was a mess, and they were supposed to have cleaned it before going out to play. I screamed at them, "Get off the goddamn bike and get in the house!" I think the neighborhood kids were more afraid than they were. I grabbed the belt and belted both of them on the legs. I've done it before, but this time God meant for me to have the lesson. As I'm belting them, I'm yelling about how they could have been hurt. "Is that what you want? To get hurt? You'll come running in the house crying after you've fallen and skinned your arms and legs." I saw it in my oldest one's eyes. She never said a thing, but her look said, What's the difference between that and what you are doing now? I was trying so hard to protect them from harm, when someone should have been protecting them from me.*

When you spank your child when she runs in front of the car, are you being the protector or are you hurting the child? Be aware of the difference.

MOM THE PROVIDER OR NURTURER

A mother feeds her children only warm, nourishing meals on a set schedule—and they eat everything.
        —Carolyn

This role is where women with anger issues hold a lot of guilt. The stereotyped mother is one who is forever nurturing and loving. It doesn't allow for women to have a human side. Most anger around this role derives from guilt. Carolyn shared her experience with her guilt and anger.

It just never seems to work out. I'm a single mother and always so busy. Just when I think I'm getting it together, something happens. I always end up grabbing something quick for breakfast, which usually means giving my kids doughnuts or sugar to start their day with. Sometimes we don't get to eat dinner until 9:00 or 10:00 P.M., and then it's fast food. By the end of the day, all three of us are so irritable from not eating or eating bad stuff and running all day. That's when all the guilt sets in, and finally just I explode. Instead of calming down for the night, we are all in turmoil. I lie in bed crying, telling myself that it's going to be different tomorrow. But then I don't get enough sleep, I wake up irritable, and it all starts over again.

Carolyn feels like she is less of a mom if she can't do it all. Unfortunately many women, like Carolyn, don't ask for help because they believe that to do so would reflect badly on them. They may fear that social services will get involved. Later in this chapter, I'll talk more about the importance of asking for help.

Do you feel guilty about not being able to provide certain things for your child? What exactly are those things that you feel you cannot provide or provide poorly?

. . . .

. . . .

. . . .

. . . .

. . . .

MOM THE ROLE MODEL

A mother never cusses or loses her temper. She always does the right thing and is willing to sacrifice for others.
—Tonya

Your child learns to deal with situations with anger by watching you. You may hope otherwise, but you know it's true. You find yourself saying the same things to your children that your mother said to you. Then you panic: *Oh no, I've become my mother!* It can be scary, but it's even scarier when you consider that you actually paid attention to what she was saying. And that means your children are paying attention to you.

It's okay to talk about your anger with your children. Being open about the issue is not letting your children see your weak side, as many women believe. Trust me, your children have already seen it. In fact, admitting you have a problem, showing you're human, looking for and working for a solution, and involving your children in a productive way are all great qualities for a good role model. Asking your children for their opinion and assistance empowers them and gives them a sense of usefulness. Here is a solution that Tonya's son came up with on his own.

My son is always acting like a clown, but many times he truly is funny. We were in the car, and I was cursing strongly at some idiot who almost caused a three-car pileup. When I took a breath from venting, my son said, "Yeah, and I hope when you get to work, you have a booger hanging out of your nose." I couldn't help but laugh. The mood changed immediately in the car. I never said anything, but I have noticed that he uses humor more and more when I get angry. And it works.

Kristi and her child came up with a different way of handling Kristi's anger.

When I get angry when we are at home, my daughter says, "I'm going to my room for a little bit." It's like a signal to me to think back to our conversation. It gives me an opportunity to not say something or do something I'll regret. It gives her a chance to not be a victim of my outrage. She's a lot more in tune to what is going on than I thought she was.

Barbara told a story about when she was in the car with her son, Justin. She had just picked him up from school after having a really bad day. Justin was wound up from playing and jumped in the car saying, "Let's go to McDonald's!" Barbara snapped, "Don't you start with me! I've had nothing but shit from people all day. I have got to find another job soon. Those bastards! Anyway, you don't need to be eating McDonald's every day! Just be quiet and don't push me." Justin replied in an unusually calm voice, "Mom, it's not my fault." It took a lot of strength for Justin to say those few words. And Barbara had to swallow a bit of pride.

What are some things your child could do or say when you are angry that would help?

. . . .

. . . .

. . . .

. . . .

. . . .

. . . .

. . . .

. . . .

. . . .

Sit down and talk with your kids about your anger. Listen to what your children say about your anger and how it affects them. Work with them to devise a plan that will help you and your children deal with anger outbursts.

MOM THE FRIEND OR CONFIDANT

A mother remains calm, clear minded, and without emotion when her child tells her that he has done something wrong.
    —Stacy

If a friend came to you with a situation at work where she made a mistake, how would you react? Would you support her, encourage her, and give her advice? Or would you lose your temper, put her down, and yell at her for being irresponsible and careless? Sometimes, we give more respect, understanding, and tolerance to a friend than we do our own children. When your child tells you he has done something wrong, he is coming to you for help. If you become angry and aggressive, you could be sending a signal that it's better not to tell anyone, that he shouldn't ask for help or support, and that he is somehow less of a person for making a mistake. If you believe that part of being a mother is being a friend, extend your child the same courtesy you would to a friend.

❧

Describe the last time you were angry with your child for making a mistake.

. . . .

. . . .

. . . .

. . . .

. . . .

. . . .

. . . .

What was the message you gave your child with your response?

. . . .

. . . .

. . . .

. . . .

. . . .

. . . .

. . . .

❧

Asking for Help

Many women believe that asking for help means they are not good mothers. I argue that a good mother knows when it's time to ask for help. Asking for help could prove to be the most powerful thing you can do. Women also fear repercussions from social services and other agencies if they seek professional help. But let's face it: the repercussions of not asking for help could be devastating.

FRIENDS AND RELATIVES

Especially if you are a single mother, you may feel like you have totally exhausted your friends and relatives by asking for favors. But they may not know everything that you are going through. Talk with them about your situation, and extend some of your assistance in return. Most importantly, you can never say thank you enough. People are always more willing to help out when they know that it's appreciated.

❖

Make a list of those people you can call on to help you out.

. . . .

. . . .

. . . .

. . . .

. . . .

Think of a few small ways that you can show them your appreciation.

. . . .

. . . .

. . . .

. . . .

. . . .

. . . .

❖

DELEGATING

Yes, it's within your rights. Your spouse or partner can take on responsibility for helping you. If they are not helping, or will not help, then there lies a bigger problem. Children are also very capable of taking on some chores that are set according to their age.

What are some of the things you need help with?

. . . .

. . . .

. . . .

. . . .

. . . .

. . . .

Could your children help you with any of these tasks?

. . . .

.   . . .

. . . .

. . . .

. . . .

Is it possible for your spouse or partner to take on some of these responsibilities? How could you shift responsibilities so that neither one of you is taking on the burden of doing everything?

. . . .

. . . .

. . . .

. . . .

. . . .

. . . .

SUPPORT GROUPS OR OUTSIDE AGENCIES

Support groups can be very powerful. I believe that working in groups can be one of the most successful ways of working through anger issues. There are also agencies available that can help you. Spending a few minutes doing some research about local opportunities and support groups could prove to reduce your stress and anger.

Get a phone book or go to the Internet, and look up "community services." Find some local organizations or hotlines that you could contact for assistance, and list them below.

. . . .

. . . .

. . . .

. . . .

. . . .

. . . .

Also list individuals from your support group or friends or relatives whom you can call to talk you down. Consider making arrangements with someone who could watch your children for a few hours while you cool off, and offer to provide the same for her.

. . . .

. . . .

. . . .

. . . .

. . . .

. . . .

. . . .

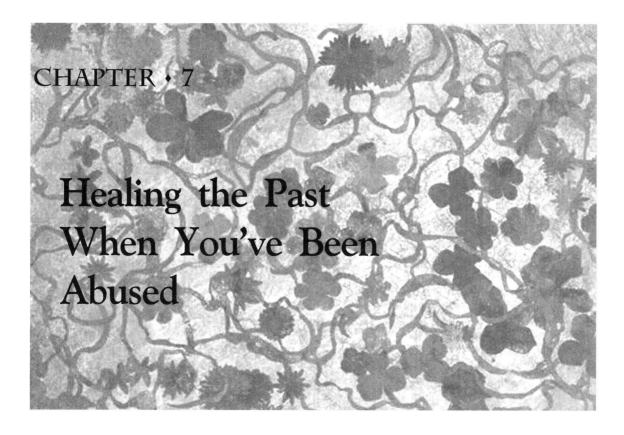

CHAPTER · 7

Healing the Past When You've Been Abused

MANY WOMEN who come into my anger management group share the painful reality of having been abused, physically, sexually, or emotionally, by family members when they were children. The most common response for these women is anger. Being abused as a child is totally unacceptable. Women have the right to feel rage at being abused. A woman's anger helps her to rise above the drowning waters of the hopelessness and depression of having been abused.

However, most women feel shame because they have misdirected their anger toward other people. It has become a destructive force, and they have lashed out at others. Many women have been shamed for their anger.

I tell each woman that first she needs to honor her anger. I'll never forget the powerful experience of telling Lonnie, a client in a group session, that I honored her anger, that her anger was not bad, that her anger had enabled her to be a survivor. She was so moved, she started crying. She said, "No one has ever said that to me before. I always thought my anger was bad. But it's not, it kept me alive. I just need to express it in a more constructive way."

Anger can actually be a positive force in the life of a woman who has been abused. This concept of anger as a healing force contradicts traditional anger management books and programs for men. Ellen Bass and Laura Davis, in *The Courage to Heal*, call anger "the backbone of healing" (1988, 315) because it keeps women going through the ups and down of the healing process. Anger can motivate you to heal, no matter what. In order for anger to work in a positive way for you, it needs to be focused at the family members who abused you.

A crucial step in understanding your anger patterns is to look back at the messages you received in the past about anger and about yourself. The exercises in this chapter will help you explore what you learned about anger from your family of origin, learn how these lessons connect to your present experience, and begin to release some of your anger in a constructive way.

How does (or did) your mother behave? How did you know when she was angry?

> *My mother would tell me she loved me one minute and then turn around and do something hurtful the next. That's how I knew she was angry with me.*
> —Linda

. . . .

. . . .

. . . .

. . . .

How does (or did) your father behave? How did you know when he was angry?

> *He used to be a major alcoholic and came home very drunk, yelling, screaming, and hollering loudly. . . . I couldn't stand it when he got drunk and rageful.*
> —Hillary

. . . .

. . . .

. . . .

. . . .

How do your brothers or sisters behave when they get angry?

> *My brother would tease me and my sister would ignore me—that's how I knew when they were angry.*
> —Jody

. . . .

. . . .

. . . .

. . . .

How do you behave when you get angry?

. . . .

. . . .

. . . .

. . . .

How did you express anger when you were little?

. . . .

. . . .

. . . .

. . . .

What messages did you get from your parents regarding your expression of anger? How did they respond to your anger?

. . . .

. . . .

. . . .

. . . .

What conclusions or decisions did you reach about anger when you were young?

. . . .

. . . .

. . . .

. . . .

How were other emotions—such as happiness and sadness—expressed in your family? Was anger the main emotion expressed in your family?

. . . .

. . . .

. . . .

. . . .

How did your parents discipline you when you were younger?

. . . .

. . . .

. . . .

. . . .

What role did you play in your family? For example, were you the family hero, clown, scapegoat, helper?

. . . .

. . . .

. . . .

. . . .

What was your family like when you were growing up?

. . . .

. . . .

. . . .

. . . .

Can you think of some words to describe your childhood?

. . . .

. . . .

. . . .

. . . .

How were anger and conflict expressed in your family (verbally, physically, or not openly expressed)?

. . . .

. . . .

. . . .

. . . .

Did your parents fight? Were the fights physical? Did you witness any violence? Did you see bruises, cuts, or other visible injuries?

. . . .

. . . .

. . . .

. . . .

Did you and your siblings fight each other? Physically?

. . . .

. . . .

. . . .

. . . .

How did your parents punish you for misbehavior? Did your parents ever hurt you physically?

. . . .

. . . .

. . . .

. . . .

❧

Using whatever art materials you have on hand, create a picture of your family of origin (the peo-ple you grew up with) and a picture of yourself in that family. Take as much time as you need. What does this picture mean to you? How did you feel making it?

❧

Look at the daily anger journal you began in chapter 3 and pick one incident from this past week when you were angry.

List three feelings you felt during or after the incident.

1. . . . .

2. . . . .

3. . . . .

Think back to a time when you were younger than fifteen and felt the same or similar feelings. Describe that experience.

. . . .

. . . .

. . . .

Describe how you would change that experience if you could go back in time.

. . . .

. . . .

. . . .

Write endings to these two sentences:

1. Turning my anger on myself has hurt me by . . . .

. . . .

2. I have misdirected my anger toward others and hurt them by . . . .

. . . .

Fear of getting angry is one of the main reasons women stop themselves from feeling anger or from directing it at those who abused them. Some women feel afraid that the anger will take over their life or that they will lose control and hurt someone.

Complete the following sentence:

I'm afraid that if I allowed myself to express my anger, ...

. . . .

. . . .

. . . .

. . . .

If you were abused in any way, write a letter to those who abused you. Let your thoughts and feelings flow; don't judge your thoughts or feelings. So that you really feel free to express yourself, write a letter you are *not* going to send. (Remember that anger is a feeling and you do not have to act on your feelings when expressing your anger about being abused. You can decide later whether you want to write a letter to send.)

The spoken or unspoken messages you received as a child from your parents, caregivers, teachers, relatives, and friends can have tremendous influence on how you feel about yourself and how you live your life. When you identify and understand the negative messages you received, you can begin to let those messages go. Positive messages can boost your self-esteem and provide inspiration.

❧

List three significant family members or caregivers and the messages you received from them. Example:

1. Mother   It is selfish to put yourself before others.

2. Father   Don't be so sure of yourself.

3. Grandma   You can do whatever you want.

1. . . . .

2. . . . .

3. . . . .

❧

As you move forward in your healing, it helps to reflect on who you are and who you would like to become. Sandra Thomas (1993) suggests that you write in your anger journal about your angry feelings toward your parents (living or not) and anyone else who is out of sight but still living rent free in your head. Letting go and making something new of your relationship with your parents or caregivers can be very healing.

Carol Tavris (1989) recommends that you create a healing ritual to mark this important occasion and honor the fact that you are beginning to let go of your anger toward your parents or caregivers. Your ritual should involve signs and symbols that are meaningful to you. For example, you might get out some old family photos, write a poem or song, paint a family portrait, or even plant a tree. Hopefully, you'll experience some emotional release as you conduct your ritual. This can also be a powerful emotional experience when you do it in a group setting.

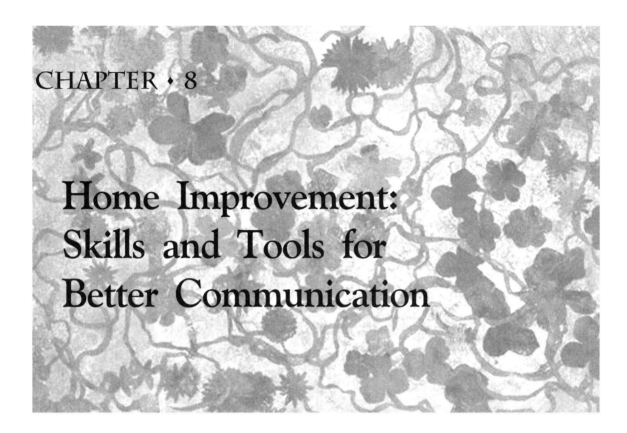

CHAPTER · 8

Home Improvement: Skills and Tools for Better Communication

THE MOST effective communication between people is direct communication of what you want, feel, see, believe, and sense. When you explain or justify what you want, most of the energy goes into the explanations, and people may not hear what you really want to communicate. You give away your power to the one to whom you are explaining. You can want something just because you want it!

I-Messages

I-messages (also called *I-statements*) are respectful statements that keep responsibility with the person giving them. With I-messages, you are sharing yourself in a nonjudgmental way, giving a gift of yourself to another person. This is in contrast to blaming, accusatory statements that begin *You always*, *You never*, or *You don't*; such statements are likely to make the listener feel defensive. Here are some examples of different kinds of respectful I-messages.

SHARING YOUR IDEAS

My point of view is . . .

It appears to me that . . .

My thinking at the present time is . . .

IDENTIFYING ISSUES

I hear you saying . . .

I want to know how you feel.

I'd like to hear what you think we should do.

ASKING FOR WHAT YOU WANT

I want to have dinner with you next Thursday.

I want a hug.

I want to work with you.

SHARING YOUR FEELINGS

I feel warm when I'm with you.

I feel free when I'm with you.

I'm glad that you invited me.

For each of the following situations, identify the feeling (or feelings) you might experience if this happened to you. Fill in the next sentence stating your needs and wants.

Your partner has been very quiet and unresponsive to you all evening, and you want some attention.

When you don't talk to me, I feel . . . .

I need/want . . . .

. . . .

. . . .

Your partner is driving too fast.

When you drive too fast, I feel . . . .

I need/want . . . .

. . . .

. . . .

Your partner is flirting with another woman.

When you flirt with her, I feel . . . .

I need/want . . . .

. . . .

. . . .

Your partner comes home for dinner two hours late without offering an explanation.

When you come home two hours late, I feel . . . .

I need/want . . . .

. . . .

. . . .

Your friend said she would come over and baby-sit, and she never showed up.

When you didn't show up to babysit, I felt . . . .

I need/want . . . .

. . . .

. . . .

Your partner keeps leaving a mess in the kitchen after you have asked him or her to clean up numerous times.

When you leave a mess, I feel . . . .

I need/want . . . .

. . . .

. . . .

Your sister criticizes the way you discipline your children.

When you criticize the way I discipline my children, I feel . . . .

I need/want . . . .

. . . .

. . . .

You had plans to go out with a friend tonight, but your partner asks you to stay home.

When you ask me to stay home, I feel . . . .

I need/want . . . .

. . . .

. . . .

❖

Problem-Solving Skills

Constructive problem solving involves effective communication skills. To communicate well, you must pay attention to what you say and to how and when you say something. Listed below are some do's and don'ts that are important to remember. I recommend that you practice these skills first when you are not in an angry situation. It is a lot harder to practice in situations when you already feel angry.

WHEN

DO make sure that both you and the other person are ready and able to talk about a problem before getting into it.

DON'T bring up something when you are walking out or leaving.

DON'T bring up your issues in response to the other person stating his or hers.

HOW

DO try to face the other person directly. Keep eye contact, and keep a relaxed and open body posture when talking.

DON'T look away, cross your arms, or clench your fists when you talk.

DO try to speak in a normal tone and at a normal pace.

DON'T shout, yell, or talk too fast or too long if you can help it.

HOW MUCH

DO keep it simple. Try to talk about just one thing at time.

DON'T give a long list of backlogged issues in a big lump.

Time-Outs

In *Dr. Weisinger's Anger Work-Out Book* (1985), Hendrie Weisinger suggests taking a *time-out* as a simple technique for getting out of a situation that might otherwise lead to abuse or unhealthy communication. Either partner in a relationship should use it when they feel angry or afraid. To use a time-out, you need to be aware of your own level of tension or "explosiveness" and to be willing to walk away when you feel that you are too angry to work out a problem.

Weisinger states what a time-out is and what it is not. A time-out is

❧   a chance for you to get away from an argument and cool down so that you can better solve the problem when you come back

❧   an opportunity to find some appropriate physical release for your anger, like walking quickly, running, shooting some hoops, doing a relaxation exercise, or imagining yourself in a calm, peaceful place

❧   a short break taken from a "hot" situation

❧   a message to your partner (or child) that you care enough about him or her to take some time to cool down

A time-out is not

❧   a chance to go out and have fun with your friends

❧   a time to watch TV, drink, do drugs, or engage in violent behavior

❧   a time to spend a day or two away from your partner

❧   a chance to say unkind or blaming things

❧   an opportunity to punish, manipulate, or control your partner

Taking time-outs can

❧   reduce violence between partners or friends

❧   reduce your need to control other people

❧   contribute to greater trust in your relationship

❧   make it possible to start solving the difficult issues and differences in your relationship

❧   increase your sense of internal control

Time-outs are to be used when you are angry and need to take a break in order to not escalate the situation. When you take a time-out, you are taking an action.

It's important to introduce the time-out concept to your partner when you're both feeling calm and you're not already in the middle of an argument. When you are introducing the concept to your partner, ask him or her to read this section of the book. Then ask for help. You could say something like, "I know I haven't been good at this in the past. If I feel that our discussion or trying to work something out isn't working, because of something I or you or both of us are doing, I need this option. The way I'll do this is to ask for a time-out, ask not to discuss the issue further at that time, and ask to arrange another time to discuss it."

It is important that you avoid power struggles by making it clear that your partner, too, can initiate a time-out. Another key point is to learn to give up having the last word; it's momentarily satisfying but never very productive. When one person takes a time-out, the other person is not allowed to follow the person out of the room. It is not okay to block someone's exit or have your exit blocked.

Let's review the steps in taking a time-out:

1. Identify how you are feeling.

2. Decide whether the situation—and the way it is making you feel—is acceptable to you. You may first try to express yourself by asking a question like, "Would you please lower your voice?" In other words, try to manage the situation, modify it, or ask for a change, and if you don't get it, ask for a time-out.

3. In asking for a time-out, you can begin by saying something like, "I'm beginning to feel anger, and I want to take a time-out."

4. You can follow that with "I'm not avoiding the issue. I will discuss this at a later time," and then proceed to set the time. If the other person doesn't get it at first, I recommend that you try this twice and then take your time-out. The time-out does not need to be okayed by the other person. A key point here is that if no later time is arranged to finish the discussion, it is the person who takes the time-out who is responsible for reapproaching their partner.

5. When the agreed-upon time is reached, the person who called the time-out states, "I'm ready to talk about this. Are you willing to talk?"

6. If the other person is not willing, then once again negotiate a time to talk.

Here are some other points to remember:

❧   The more you feel the need to engage and talk with your partner, the more important it is that you *don't.*

❧   Pick one issue, not a whole backlog of complaints.

❧   Stress what you want—not what you don't want—from your partner.

❧   Make your requests in a positive way, otherwise it will lead to resentment.

❧   Keep in mind that you don't have to resolve every issue in one sitting.

Over the next week, try to use time-outs in situations that make you feel angry. Then, in the spaces below, list two examples of what happened when you took a time-out.

Situation:

. . . .

. . . .

. . . .

. . . .

Results:

. . . .

. . . .

. . . .

. . . .

Situation:

. . . .

. . . .

. . . .

. . . .

Results:

. . . .

. . . .

. . . .

. . . .

Communication Styles: Aggressive, Passive, and Assertive

In this section, we'll look at three communication styles. Each style involves a particular verbal and nonverbal approach to communication, and each style has a unique impact on other people.

AGGRESSIVE COMMUNICATION

When you communicate aggressively, you express your opinion in a way that violates the rights of others. Humiliation, sarcasm, insults, and power are often used. The goal of aggression is domination and winning, forcing the other person to lose. The basic messages are

This is what I think. You are stupid for believing differently.

This is what I want. What you want is not important.

This is what I feel. Your feelings don't count.

NONASSERTIVE OR PASSIVE COMMUNICATION

When you communicate passively or nonassertively, you give in to other people's requests, demands, or feelings without regard to what you want or feel. Being nonassertive or passive often violates your rights. Because you fail to express honest feelings, thoughts, and beliefs, you permit others to violate you. If you express your feelings in an apologetic, timid, or self-effacing manner, others can easily disregard them. The message is *I don't count. You can take advantage of me.* It shows a lack of respect for your own needs. The goal of nonassertion is to avoid conflict at any cost.

ASSERTIVE COMMUNICATION

Assertive communication involves standing up for your personal rights and expressing thoughts and beliefs in direct, honest, and appropriate ways that do not violate the other's rights. Your message expresses who you are, and you convey it without dominating, humiliating, or degrading the other person. Assertiveness involves respect—not deference. The goal of assertion is communication and mutuality; that is, to get and give respect, to ask for fair play, and to leave room for compromise when the needs and rights of two people conflict. In such compromises, neither person sacrifices basic integrity, and both get some of their needs satisfied.

Passive-Assertive-Aggressive Styles Chart

	Passive	Assertive	Aggressive
Intent of your actions is to	• Hide your feelings • Deny yourself • Avoid conflicts • Avoid risks and stay out of trouble • Avoid hurting or disappointing others • Be liked at all costs	• Express your feelings • Communicate with others • Show respect for self/others • Be direct and honest • Stand up for your rights • Achieve your goals	• Strongly express your feelings • Set others straight • Do it your way • Disregard others • "Win" • Achieve your goals regardless of means
Nonverbal or stylistic aspects of behavior	• Lack of eye contact • Soft voice level • Hesitant speech • Weak or helpless gestures • Slumped posture	• Direct eye contact • Conversational voice level • Confident, fluent speech • Firm but controlled gestures • Erect posture	• Glaring eye contact • Loud voice level • Fast, pressured speech • Threatening gestures • Intimidating or "closed" posture
Likely reactions of others	Others often believe • Your feelings or opinions aren't important • You have little or nothing to offer • You are a pushover Others are likely to • Not take you seriously • Ignore you • Manipulate or abuse you	Others often believe • You are up front with your feelings • You are prepared to defend your rights • You have self-respect and confidence Others are likely to • Take you seriously • Listen to you • Take your needs or opinions into account	Others often believe • You are too pushy • You are insensitive and rude • You are a "crazy" or unpleasant person Others are likely to • Resent or dislike you • Become angry, hostile, or uncooperative in return • Avoid you

Adapted from *Responsible Assertive Behavior, Cognitive/Behavioral Procedures for Trainers*, by Arthur J. Lange and Patricia Jakubowski. Champaign, Illinois: Research Press, 1976.

Look back at the daily anger journal you started in chapter 3. Write down situations from your own experience that are examples of each communication style.

Passive:

. . . .

. . . .

. . . .

. . . .

Assertive:

. . . .

. . . .

. . . .

. . . .

Aggressive:

. . . .

. . . .

. . . .

. . . .

❦

Read each of the following situations and pick the response that best describes you.

1. Your partner was going to meet you at 5:00 P.M. and shows up at 5:45 P.M. without offering an explanation. How would you respond?

  a. Not say anything, but sulk for a while.

  b. Say, "I'm disappointed that you're late, and I would like to know why you didn't call."

  c. Say, "It's about time! You're always late! You are so inconsiderate. Why didn't you call?"

2. Your friend asks to borrow some money from you. How would you respond?

  a. Go ahead and lend the money, secretly hoping you'll get paid back.

  b. Say no.

  c. Say, "I don't have any money to lend."

3. You and your partner were planning to spend a quiet evening alone together. Your partner wants to go over to a friend's house instead. How do you respond?

    a. Say, "I'm disappointed. I wanted to spend the evening alone with you."

    b. Say, "Okay, whatever you want to do."

    c. Say, "You always do this to me! I'm sick of being second! Forget you!"

4. Your partner wants to have sex and you don't want to. How would you respond?

    a. Don't say anything and just go along with it to avoid a conflict.

    b. Say, "I wish just once we could cuddle together without it leading to sex."

    c. Say, "I really don't feel in the mood right now."

5. You have received an unfair evaluation from your boss. You feel you should have received a better evaluation. How would you respond?

    a. Part of you thinks that the boss might be right, and you feel like a failure.

    b. You decide the boss is a jerk and complain to your coworkers.

    c. You talk with your boss and say, "I disagree with my evaluation."

6. Your sister asks you to babysit her two children on Saturday. You had planned to have a relaxing day to yourself. How would you respond?

    a. Say, "Sis, I really want the day to myself," and hope she backs off.

    b. Say, "Okay, I guess so," and feel resentful.

    c. Say, "I think you're too dependent on me."

ASSERTIVENESS BILL OF RIGHTS

Here are some fundamental rights based on the idea of assertiveness. These are adapted from Manuel Smith's 1975 book, *When I Say No I Feel Guilty*.

    ❧ I have the right to have and express my own feelings and opinions, and to experience the consequences.

    ❧ I have the right to judge my own behavior, thoughts, and emotions and to take responsibility for their initiation and consequences upon myself.

    ❧ I have the right to offer no reasons or excuses justifying my behavior and to accept the consequences of my behavior.

    ❧ I have the right to change my mind.

    ❧ I have the right to make mistakes and be responsible for them.

    ❧ I have the right to set my own priorities.

❖　I have the right to ask for what I want.

❖　I have the right to choose not to assert myself.

❖　I have the right to get what I pay for.

❖　I have the right to ask for information from professionals.

❖　I have the right to say *no*, *I don't know*, and *I don't understand.*

❖　I have the responsibility to recognize that everyone else has these same rights.

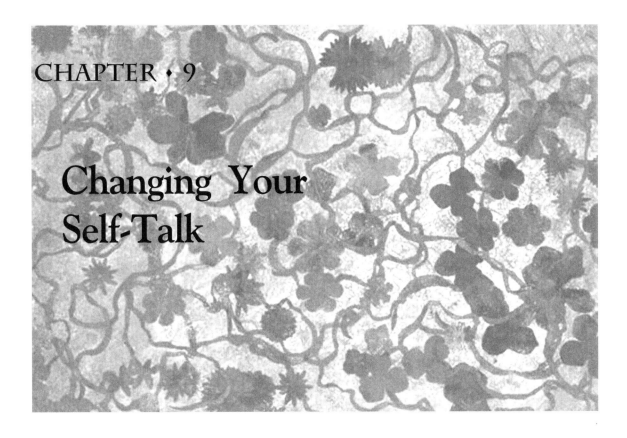

CHAPTER · 9

Changing Your Self-Talk

SELF-STATEMENTS (Beck 1976) are messages we develop over time to explain the world and how we fit into it. We have statements about ourselves as women; as wives, partners, and girlfriends; as homemakers; as mothers; as friends; as workers; as daughters; and in all kinds of other roles. We develop most of our statements as children.

Self-statements often include a "should." "Shoulds," when we use them, usually refer to the rules of life. For example, we have rules like *I should not steal; I should be respectful of older people; Women should be kind and understanding; Good wives should cook dinner for their husbands; Good mothers should have well-behaved children;* and thousands more.

As adults, we learn there really are few rules in life but many choices. If I believe I should not steal and my family is starving, I may choose to steal rather than let them die. A that point, my "should" becomes a choice.

When the word *should* comes up in your vocabulary, you are probably quoting a rule you learned before age eight. Your perspective in the world at eight is very different from what it is now that you're an adult. Self-statements don't grow up. They can, however, be changed if you want to change them.

According to Beck, there are three main kinds of self-statements.

BELIEFS OR "SHOULDS." We usually learn these when we are children, from our parents, other family members, teachers, and real and fictional childhood heroes.

Example: A man should always be the family breadwinner.

INTERPRETATIONS OF EVENTS. We interpret everything that happens to us according to our own subjective point of view, which is not always accurate.

Example: A coworker walks by and doesn't answer when you say hi. You assume that he is unfriendly or has an attitude. The fact of the matter is that his mother just had a stroke and he is too upset to pay attention to what's going on around him. Because you don't know what his story is, you get angry with him. Your interpretation is that he is being unfriendly. If you knew the facts of the situation, you would interpret it differently.

SELF-TALK. We talk to ourselves about situations and tell ourselves how to react based on what we have learned in the past.

Example: You stub your toe on a chair that is not in its usual place. You feel pain, but you learned early on that you shouldn't express pain, so you say to yourself, *It's my husband's fault. He should have put the chair back where it belongs.*

When you find yourself getting angry this next week, ask yourself:

What beliefs do I have about this situation that is causing me to get angry?

. . . .

. . . .

. . . .

What is my interpretation of this event? Is it accurate?

. . . .

. . . .

. . . .

How am I talking to myself? Is my self-talk triggering my anger, or is it helping me to feel calmer?

. . . .

. . . .

. . . .

Negative Self-Talk and Anger

Negative self-talk contributes to anger. You may start out feeling just a little bit angry about something that happened, but the more you think about it, the angrier you get. Negative self-talk includes blaming other people for the way you feel, labeling other people as bad, or interpreting other people's actions as intentional.

Remembering all the "bad" things another person did to you and building a case against the other person makes things worse than they are. When you become excessively angry, you experience stress. As a result, you may not think or speak effectively. In fact, you may even think or speak words that do not give an accurate picture of what is going on. Beck and Emery (1985) call this "cognitive distortion."

Certain words exaggerate or overstate how bad a problem really is. The use of such extreme words leads to inaccurate perceptions and unfair demands. It's a good idea to learn to recognize these key words and use them as cues to rephrase your speaking and thinking:

always	*awful*	*should*	*must*
never	*terrible*	*ought*	*have to*
forever	*can't stand*	*unfair*	*no right*

Here's how it works: A series of good, bad, and neutral events happen to you. You filter this input through your own beliefs, interpretations, and past experiences. The end product is your thoughts and feelings. Very often, your style of thinking determines how you see the world and how you feel about the world and about yourself. When you have a feeling that's intense, try to find out the thoughts that helped to create it.

Negative self-talk comes in several different varieties:

ALL-OR-NOTHING THINKING. *That guy is always a pain in the ass!* or *I never do anything right.*

OVERGENERALIZATION. *Nothing ever goes right. My life is so miserable.*

JUMPING TO CONCLUSIONS. This kind of cognitive distortion comes in two types: mind reading (*I bet my boss is going to ask me to work overtime again*) and fortune telling (*She won't call me—I just know it*).

BINOCULAR TRICKS. This involves making mountains out of molehills, or molehills out of mountains. Binocular tricks include magnification (*I hate it when you're late—I hate having to always wait for you*) and minimization (*Oh, don't worry about it, it's nothing, really*).

EMOTIONAL REASONING. *I'm angry at you. You're trying to provoke me so I'll get arrested.*

"SHOULD" STATEMENTS. *He has no right!* or *She shouldn't cry over him, he's not worth it.*

LABELING AND MISLABELING. *I'm a loser* or *He's a dog.*

PERSONALIZATION. *Everyone I try to talk to ignores me. It must be my fault.*

❦

What kind of cognitive distortions do you use?

. . . .

. . . .

. . . .

. . . .

. . . .

. . . .

. . . .

❦

Positive Self-Talk

Positive self-talk can help you stay calm or control your anger when it comes up.

❦

Below is a list of situations and a positive self-statement to go with each situation. Add your own positive self-statement to each of the situations listed below.

Someone cuts in front of you on the freeway.

❦   *I don't have to get angry.*

❦   . . . .

Your partner is ten minutes late.

❦   *I can choose to stay calm if I want to.*

❦   . . . .

Your coworker wants to talk to you about something at work.

❦   *I don't need to feel threatened here.*

❦   . . . .

You're stuck in traffic.

❧   *I can relax and let go of my anger.*

❧   . . . .

Your child just spilled milk all over the floor.

❧   *I am in control of my own emotions.*

❧   . . . .

It's been raining all day, and you were going to have a picnic outside.

❧   *I'm not going to allow things outside of me to control what goes on inside of me.*

❧   . . . .

The driver in front of you keeps stepping on her brakes.

❧   *I feel upset, but I know how to deal with it.*

❧   . . . .

Your husband forgot it was your anniversary.

❧   *I am responsible for taking care of my own needs.*

❧   . . . .

You're angry with your husband for forgetting your anniversary.

❧   *I know how to express my feelings without getting abusive.*

❧   . . . .

Your ex-husband did not drop off the kids on time.

❧   *I can't control other people.*

❧   . . . .

You're angry at your ex-husband for not dropping off the kids on time.

❧   *I can only control myself and how I express my feelings.*

❧   . . . .

The driver in the car next to you just flipped you off.

❧   *If this person wants to go off on me, that's her problem.*

❧   . . . .

A pedestrian yells at you for driving too close to him.

❧   *I don't need to respond by being angry.*

❧   . . . .

A newspaper reporter writes a negative story about you.

❧   *No matter what other people say, I believe in myself.*

❧   . . . .

Your landlord is upset because the rent is late.

❧   *I'm the only person who can make me mad or keep me calm.*

❧   . . . .

The people next to you in the restaurant are talking loudly.

❧   *People are going to act the way they want to, not the way I want them to act.*

❧   . . . .

You are about to go into your boss's office for a performance review.

❧   *I know that I can handle this well.*

❧   . . . .

❧

Attitudes

Attitudes are an emotional response to people, places, and situations. We are not born with attitudes; we learn them from our relationships with our friends and parents, and from the outcome of our past experiences. We continue to learn as we grow older, but we may not be aware that we have become conditioned to feel, think, and act in certain ways.

Anger may have clouded your thinking with resentment, fear, and self-pity. It is an important part of healing to change your attitudes. You must be willing to learn new ways of feeling comfortable with yourself and others. One way to begin to do this is by examining your attitudes.

❧

Give an example of a tool you use to let go of the past and focus on today.

. . . .

. . . .

Describe a situation when you avoided judging another person's motives and behavior.

. . . .

. . . .

. . . .

. . . .

Describe how you kept the focus on yourself.

. . . .

. . . .

. . . .

. . . .

Think of an event that happened recently, one you had no control over, and describe how you chose a positive attitude in response to it.

. . . .

. . . .

. . . .

. . . .

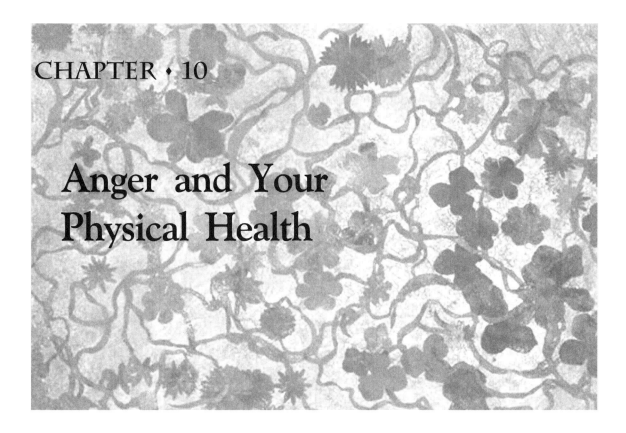

CHAPTER · 10

Anger and Your Physical Health

WHILE THE research is clear that anger increases when stress levels are high, it is not as clear regarding anger and women's health. Women who deny their anger or who experience a lot of anger are at risk of cardiovascular illness, headaches, and stomachaches (Emerson and Harrison 1990). Like most of us, when you're angry, you probably have one particular part of your body that bears the brunt of your anger. Jeannie explains the pain in her stomach when she feels angry:

> *My stomach gets tied up in knots. I get a sick feeling, especially when the initial anger occurs, until I have time to deal with that a little and try to calm myself down.*

Leslie's colon was the site of her anger:

> *I had so much anger. I really didn't know why I had the spastic colon. I was in constant pain. I just kept all my anger in, and it almost destroyed my colon.*

Instead of a specific place in her body, Rachel's whole body was being severely affected by her suppressed anger:

> *I've always tried to suppress my anger and not become explosive, because I'm afraid people will reject me or won't like me. Everything inside me was messed up because of it.*

Or maybe you're more like Jody:

My anger takes the form of headaches and neck aches. It hurts a lot when I get them. I ended up taking a lot of Advil to try and kill the pain, not realizing what I needed to do was deal with my anger instead!

Women who deny their anger are also at risk for asthma, arthritis, elevated blood pressure, insomnia, ulcers, back pain, and obesity (Munhall 1992). Rates of diagnosed breast cancer were found to be high in women who openly expressed their anger and also in those women who displayed frequent outbursts, compared to women who exhibited fewer anger outbursts (Thomas 1993). Anger is sometimes changed into a physical symptom, in what Munhall (1992, 485) calls a "socially accepted pathology," while the anger itself remains unacknowledged and therefore is not addressed. The assesment below, reprinted with permission from *Staying Young* by Tom Monte, will help you evaluate whether anger is affecting your health.

Anger-Related Health Issues Assessment
    Circle yes or no for each statement below.

   1. I have frequent headaches (or other aches and pains).   Yes   No

   2. I have abnormally high blood pressure.   Yes   No

   3. I seldom talk about my anger, even when I feel like it.   Yes   No

   4. I smoke cigarettes.   Yes   No

   5. My use of over-the-counter drugs is high.   Yes   No

   6. I have trouble letting go of things that upset me.   Yes   No

   7. I weigh more than the amount that is appropriate for me.   Yes   No

   8. I have trouble getting enough sleep.   Yes   No

   9. I drink alcoholic beverages to unwind and relax.   Yes   No

  10. My future doesn't look too bright.   Yes   No

  11. I have fewer friends now than I did a year ago.   Yes   No

  12. I don't get enough exercise.   Yes   No

  13. I know my stress level is too high.   Yes   No

If you have more than three or four yes answers, take a good look at how your anger is taking a toll on your physical health. For example, if you have recurrent headaches or neck aches, is anger hitting you on your head or neck? Or, if you have colitis, is unexpressed anger eating you up? Is your hidden anger contributing to your sleeplessness, back trouble, or being a couch potato? Whatever the case is, listen to your physical symptoms to hear what they're saying. Symptoms are one way your body is giving you a clue to tell you that something isn't right. Once you stop covering up your angry feelings with cigarettes or food, you can make the connection between anger and food and see what's really eating at you.

The denial or suppression of anger is also related to psychosomatic symptoms such as backaches, anxiety, fear, and panic attacks. The indirect expression of anger through obscenity, rudeness, and hostility has also been linked as a risk factor for heart disease (Thomas 1993). Studies have also found a link between poor health habits and anger expression. Modcrin-McCarthy and Tollet (1993) found that women who hold anger in or express it somatically (through body symptoms such as back pain and headaches) had poor self-care habits. They suggest that these women are tired, unhealthy, and unfit, and too angry to care.

How Anger Can Lead to Eating Disorders

Although several studies have looked at the link between overeating and emotions, few studies have examined anger specifically or focused exclusively on women. According to Russell and Shirk (1993, 181), emotions that were a response to "injustice, resentment, discrimination, and rejection" triggered anger in women. The researchers identified food as a woman's drug of choice. My client Maggie relates her view:

Food is my drug of choice. It's so easily accessible. And it's legal! I'll never get busted for having a burger and fries!

Russell and Shirk concluded that binge eating in response to feeling anger was a contributing factor in obesity in women. Arnow, Kenardy, and Agras (1992) found that women experienced negative emotions before and after bingeing. Any relief from anger (among other feelings) that bingeing offered, however, was temporary. My client Keri explains her cycle:

When I get mad at my husband, I'll have a slice of pizza or two and eat it as fast as I can. If I'm angry at my children, I find myself bingeing in the middle of the night. Instead of getting angry at them, I eat all of my angry feelings away. The problem is, the feelings only go away for a little while, but the weight I've gained from all the food I've eaten remains.

Whether it was Hostess Twinkies, Sara Lee cheesecake, or Häagen-Dazs ice cream, many of us learned about comfort food in the crib. Indeed, food is often the first source of comfort and love women receive. Regardless of the cause of our emotional distress, many of us still soothe ourselves with food.

Some feminist researchers explain that our one-down position as women—subordinate to fathers, husbands, and bosses—compels us to "stuff" our anger, that is, to literally stuff ourselves with food rather than express our anger or disagreement. Woodman (1980) found overeating to be present in all of the women she studied. These women rarely expressed rage. Henrietta, a participant in one of my anger management groups, used food as a way to stuff her anger and then purged it as a way to cleanse herself of anger.

The way I coped with angry feelings was with food. I would eat to make myself feel better. I've been a compulsive eater since I was a young girl. I felt helpless when I was angry because I didn't feel like I had any right to express it. So, by forcing myself to throw up, it was a way of getting my anger out of me.

After years of stuffing our anger, many of us have paid a high physical price. We're overweight, we're tired more often, we exercise less, and then we get mad at ourselves for ending up this way. This vicious cycle sends us back to the kitchen for more. Margaret knows this cycle well:

Being overweight, I get angry at myself for the shape my body is in. I used to work out and was fit. I'll go on a diet for a while, but then my feelings get the better of me, and I go off and binge again. And then I feel discouraged, like, what's the use?

Reclaiming Your Health

In the remainder of this chapter, we'll look at three important approaches to protecting your physical health: healthy eating, physical exercise, and healthy expression of anger.

HEALTHY EATING

If you are concerned about your weight, start by talking to your primary care provider. Then, take a long look at your emotionally motivated eating patterns. One way you can work toward the goal of binge-free eating is to start looking at your anger patterns. Use your anger journal to record episodes in which you ate in response to being angry, and be sure to write down what you've eaten.

Next, you need to develop healthy alternatives to angry eating, such as calling a friend before putting the food in your mouth, going for a walk, or meditating. One useful technique is just to take a deep breath. It's amazing how breathing helps you feel full. Here are some other suggestions from Thomas and Jefferson (1996):

❖   Sip water or other cool, caffeine-free beverages.

❖   If you're in anger-food crisis, talk it over with a friend. Better yet, arrange to get together.

❖   Do a household chore you've been avoiding. A lot of women say their house gets really clean when they are really mad!

❖   Do some self-care: take a bubble bath, go for a walk, or get a manicure.

❖   Use your anger energy to get something accomplished.

❖   Analyze the anger incident. Make a plan to solve the problem or react differently in the future (by asserting yourself or removing yourself from the situation, for example).

PHYSICAL EXERCISE

First, start with a physical checkup from your health-care provider. Then, make a commitment to a friend or family member (or your group, if you are working with one) to keep up the exercise program that you decide on. Making a commitment only to yourself usually doesn't bear much fruit. Keep your exercise program simple and doable, otherwise you'll quit before you even start!

I know, I know. Just the phrase itself makes you want to lie down. But if you want to improve your mental and physical health and reverse the toll that anger takes, exercise is a very helpful tool indeed.

Developing a Fitness Program

You don't have to join a gym or buy a lot of expensive workout clothes. Getting started is usually the hardest part, so be gentle with yourself. Here are some simple ways to start:

❧ Walking is just as good as running, if not better. Walking with someone or taking an exercise class together is usually more motivating than doing it alone.

❧ Get outside! I tell myself that my dogs need to go for a walk, even though I probably need to just as much as they do. They like it, and it gets me outdoors and moving.

❧ Do flexibility and stretching exercises. I keep a big yoga ball downstairs, and when I get up from working, I automatically do a backbend over it, and it helps keep me flexible and energized.

❧ Do sit-ups or push-ups, or, if you have them, work with weights.

❧ Do daily "miniworkouts" (housework, vacuuming, or walking up the stairs at work instead of taking the elevator). Every little step helps. Remember, easy does it!

Whatever program or routine you choose, make sure it's something you enjoy. If exercising is pleasurable to you, you'll be more likely to stick with it. The important thing is to keep moving, whatever it is you are doing.

Record your progress in the chart below. Try to do some kind of exercise every day.

Exercise	Mon	Tue	Wed	Thu	Fri	Sat	Sun

HEALTHY EXPRESSION OF ANGER

If you suppress your anger, your body will tell you in symptoms that something is not right. This tendency to suppress anger may be why women end up with more health problems than men. Women of all ages report more health problems and doctor visits than men, and although women live longer, women spend their later years with more chronic health conditions (Thomas 1993). Is it worth compromising your physical health to continue suppressing your anger?

Learning how to disagree is essential to clear the air. It is hard to love someone if there is conflict between you. Often, we get into arguments when we are hungry, angry, lonely, or tired. Arguments can wait. Healthy adults know that they can put arguments off until the next day or until Saturday morning. It doesn't always feel good to wait, but it is often better. As someone once said in a twelve-step program, "If it's after 10:00 P.M. and it seems like a good idea to bring something up, it's not!"

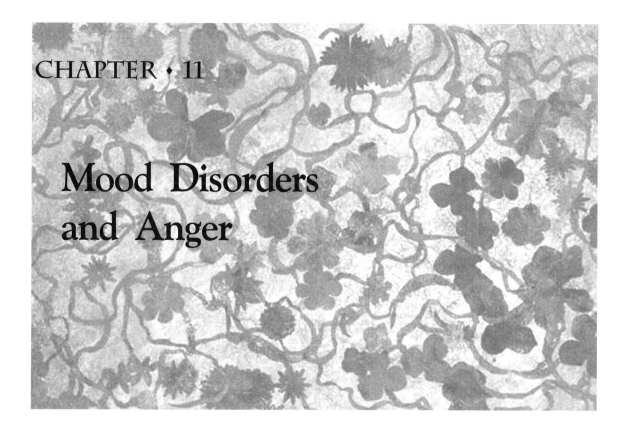

CHAPTER ♦ 11

Mood Disorders and Anger

A MOOD disorder may be temporary or permanent, depending on the circumstances, and occurs when a person loses control of their normal range of emotions. There are many known mood disorders; this book will only cover the three most common mood disorders that may affect women with anger problems. Certain mood disorders—including premenstrual syndrome, depression, and bipolar disorder—can contribute to anger problems. This chapter will help you understand each of these disorders better. I have included a self-test for each disorder so that you may become aware of a mood disorder problem, should it exist. It is important to examine your own behavior with respect to these conditions, because anger is a common denominator in depression, premenstrual syndrome, and bipolar disorder, and it would be ineffective to try to resolve only anger issues if another condition is a contributing factor.

Premenstrual Syndrome

Some women notice that they feel particularly tense, moody, irritable, or angry prior to their menstrual period. Hormone fluctuations can cause physical and emotional changes in some women. Breast tenderness, water retention, headaches, irritability, anger, depression, anxiety, and food cravings are some of the symptoms women may experience. This cluster of symptoms is called *premenstrual syndrome,* or PMS.

No one really knows what causes PMS, why some women have it and others do not, or whether it is really a syndrome at all. Regardless of these questions, many women report that they are more prone to anger when they are premenstrual (Thomas and Jefferson 1996).

> *When I am premenstrual, I have a shorter temper.*
> —Gwen

> *When I am premenstrual and tired, I am more likely to react in an angry way.*
> —Melody

> *I usually overreact with anger when I am premenstrual.*
> —Pamela

When a woman is under stress, her PMS intensifies. Stress-reduction and self-care techniques can help to alleviate PMS symptoms. Physical exercise has been found to be particularly helpful in relieving the symptoms of PMS. Walking, bicycling, swimming, or any other form of exercise performed at least three times a week can help to improve PMS.

Diet has also been found to affect the occurrence and intensity of PMS. Changes in nutrition, particularly during the two weeks before your period, can reduce or eliminate PMS symptoms. Lauersen and Stukane (1983) share the following dietary guidelines for improving PMS:

- Reduce your intake of refined sugar to five teaspoonfuls or less a day. Eliminate candy, chocolate, cake, and other desserts.

- Reduce your salt intake to less than three grams a day. Eliminate salty and pickled foods.

- Sharply reduce or eliminate your caffeine intake.

- Eliminate your alcohol intake.

- Increase your intake of complex carbohydrates (such as vegetables, whole grains, and nuts). These should be 50 to 60 percent of your diet.

- Decrease your intake of dairy products, especially cheese.

- Restrict your intake of red meat to less than three ounces a day.

- Increase your consumption of green leafy vegetables and cereals.

The B vitamins, particularly B_6, are beneficial to women suffering from PMS. Foods high in B vitamins include cereals and grains, soybeans, unsalted nuts, green leafy vegetables, rice bran, brown rice, liver, yeast, and whole-wheat bread. Good sources of vitamin B_6 include bananas, avocados, green leafy vegetables, green peppers, carrots, brewer's yeast, beef liver, whole-wheat bread, halibut, oranges, sweet potatoes, and peas. Some women find taking a B-complex vitamin helps reduce symptoms of PMS. It is, however, important to consult with a physician or nutritionist before taking more than the recommended daily allowance of any vitamin.

If you think you have PMS, begin by seeing a gynecologist for a medical evaluation. Keeping a three-month calendar of your symptoms is helpful in evaluating whether you have PMS.

Which of the following emotional, behavioral, and physical symptoms do you suffer from?

o Depression

o Irritability

o Continuous feeling of anger

o Mood swings

o Weight gain

o Breast tenderness

o Water retention

Depression: Another Face of Anger

Many women who are depressed are also angry. Depression has become a common condition in U.S. society today, and Prozac has come to be seen as our savior. Why are so many people depressed? Elevated stress levels over a sustained period of time eventually cause a physical deterioration in the areas of the brain that secrete the chemical *serotonin*. Serotonin is the substance that allows us to feel motivated and energetic. It allows us to concentrate, focus, and feel positive emotions. When we live in a complicated and stress-ridden society, our brains may become stressed, and our serotonin levels may be diminished. The behavioral results are apathy, lethargy, change in sleeping or eating habits, irritability, and sometimes anger. There are many people who are aware of their depression but don't feel they have an anger problem; you must understand that depression is also commonly thought of as anger turned inward. In simpler terms, that means anger that is repressed and not expressed.

Below is a list of common symptoms of depression. If you have five or more of these symptoms, you are probably suffering from depression and should talk with a therapist or your family doctor about treatment.

Common symptoms include:

o Difficulty concentrating

o Self-criticism

o Thoughts of hurting yourself

o Feelings of sadness and failure

o Low self-confidence

o Withdrawal and loss of interest in others

o Lack of pleasure and enjoyment

o Loss of energy

o Disturbed sleep

o Loss of appetite or increased appetite

o Wanting to stay in bed

o Feeling unattractive

Depression can lead to a cycle of ever-worsening thoughts and feelings, which can result in withdrawal and isolation. The strategy is to intervene at the level of thoughts, feelings, and/or behavior to interrupt this cycle. If you feel you are suffering from depression, you *can* be helped. The first step is to see a therapist or family doctor who can refer you, if necessary, to the appropriate specialist.

> *I found the depression symptom checklist extremely helpful in giving me insight into those "automatic" negative thoughts, but the only truly effective way for me to blast away the depression was to tackle the biochemical component in this body of mine and take antidepressant medication as well.*
> —Anna

Bipolar Disorder

A woman with anger control issues may have an underlying bipolar disorder and not even be aware of it. Bipolar disorder, also known as manic depression, affects at least 2 million Americans at any given time (Sells and Loosen 2000). The disorder is characterized by alternating periods of extreme moods. A woman with bipolar disorder experiences cycling moods that usually swing from elation, irritability, or anger (mania), to sadness and hopelessness (depression) and then back again, with periods of normal mood in between. For women who have this disorder, it can be extremely distressing and disruptive. The frequency of the swings between these two states, and the duration of the mood, varies from woman to woman.

A woman's family history and genetics often play an important role in determining the likelihood that she will have this disorder in her lifetime. Bipolar disorder typically begins in adolescence or early adulthood and continues throughout life. It is often not recognized at first as a serious disorder, and women who have it may suffer needlessly for years. This disorder is not a character flaw, and it is not your fault. It is a serious mood disorder that affects a woman's ability to function in everyday activities. It affects a woman's work, family, and social life.

Much more is known today about the causes and treatment of this mental health problem. We know that there are biological and psychological components to every bipolar disorder and that the best form of treatment is a combination of medication and psychotherapy. Bipolar disorder can be effectively managed, and a woman with the disorder can lead a normal life.

Increased stress and inadequate coping mechanisms to deal with that stress may contribute to both bipolar disorder and anger control problems. Bipolar disorder is most often experienced as a swing between a manic and a depressed mood, which may often be related to increased stress or anger. Nearly anything can trigger a woman to shift from one mood to the other, and sometimes there is no obvious trigger at all. Often, the first manic episode is triggered by some external stressor. Once a woman's mood begins to cycle, there is usually not an external reason she can find for feeling the way that she does. Because bipolar disorder and anger are so closely linked, a woman who has untreated bipolar disorder will find it very difficult to gain control of her anger.

Bipolar Symptoms Checklist

- Feeling very irritable or quick to anger

- Not feeling the need for as much sleep as you normally get

- Having thoughts that race out of control so your speech can't keep up with them

- Being distracted easily by noise or lights

- Acting overly ambitious

- Going on shopping sprees (when you don't have the money) or driving recklessly

If you have three or more of the above symptoms, you should talk to a mental health professional about whether you might have bipolar disorder. If you do have it, there are different types of treatment. With proper treatment you will be able to cope with your anger in a healthy way.

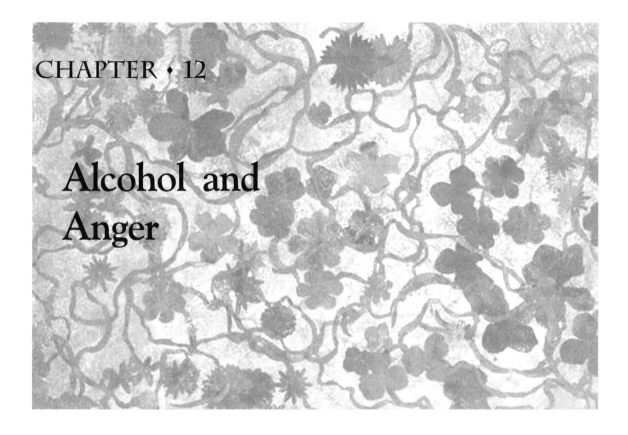

CHAPTER ♦ 12

Alcohol and Anger

A CLIENT once told me that she drank a lot in order to get rid of her anger; she feared that she would be yelling at her family all the time otherwise. But the idea that you can get rid of anger by drinking is nothing but a damaging myth, one that is all too commonly shared by people who have anger problems and drink alcohol to escape their feelings. This chapter offers you a chance to debunk your own myths, take the blinders off, and really look at the effect alcohol has, not only on your anger but on your entire life. If you are willing to take this step, you may become enlightened and see how alcohol contributed to some or even all of your anger problems. But while curbing the use of alcohol is definitely a step in the right direction, don't expect this sudden action to erase all the resentments and anger you have built up inside of you. More on that later.

How Alcohol Really Works

Alcohol is frequently mistaken for—and used as—a stress-reducer, and while this may be true in a very temporal sense, the fact is, alcohol is a central nervous system depressant which significantly affects your decision-making ability and lowers your inhibitions, thereby increasing the likelihood of irritability and outbursts of anger. Alcohol incites anger by short-circuiting the centers of the brain that control impulsive behavior and improper judgment. Ironic as all this may seem, statistics verify that approximately 55 percent of women with anger problems reported that alcohol actually escalated their anger (Hamberger 1991).

Let's clarify the effect of alcohol on emotions even further and consider what is really responsible for your anger and your angry behavior. Neither alcohol nor anger stands alone; they work together to form a synergistic combination that equals more than the sum of its parts. Alcohol may contribute to angry and aggressive behavior, but it does not cause anger. Women choose to act out their anger, just as they choose other behaviors, and while terrible choices are made under the influence of alcohol, they are still choices nonetheless. Alcohol does not force you to become angry; it triggers the emotions beneath the surface and merely allows you to suffer a lapse of reason, during which others around you may suffer the wrath of your indiscretion.

Examining Your Relationship with Alcohol

The following exercise, reprinted from *It Will Never Happen to Me* by Claudia Black (1981), will help you clarify whether you have a drinking problem. If you finish the questionnaire and discover that you really have a problem with alcohol, you may suddenly feel overwhelmed by the realization that one problem you were trying to deal with—anger—suddenly mushroomed into another problem that you were completely unaware of.

This happens to most people seeking help for just about any problem imaginable. Why is this so? Because problems don't occur in a single linear fashion, nor do we live a vacuum-sealed existence. Cause and effect, Pandora's box, Murphy's Law, and taking your car to the mechanic for one problem and finding out there are actually three more immediate and expensive problems to fix as well: these are examples of the complexity of nature and society and how everything is always related to something else. Nothing ever happens by itself.

Are You an Alcoholic?

To answer this, ask yourself the following questions and answer them honestly.

1. Do you lose time from work due to drinking?   Yes   No

2. Is drinking making your home life unhappy?   Yes   No

3. Do you drink because you are shy with other people?   Yes   No

4. Is drinking affecting your reputation?   Yes   No

5. Have you ever felt remorse after drinking?   Yes   No

6. Have you gotten into financial difficulties due to drinking?   Yes   No

7. Do you turn to lower companions and an inferior environment when drinking?
   Yes   No

8. Does your drinking make you careless of your family's welfare?   Yes   No

9. Has your ambition decreased since drinking?   Yes   No

10. Do you crave a drink at a definite time daily?   Yes   No

11. Do you want a drink the next morning?   Yes   No

12. Does drinking cause you to have difficulty in sleeping?   Yes   No

13. Has your efficiency decreased since drinking?   Yes   No

14. Is drinking jeopardizing your job or business?   Yes   No

15. Do you drink to escape from worries or troubles?   Yes   No

16. Do you drink alone?   Yes   No

17. Have you ever had a complete loss of memory as a result of drinking?   Yes   No

18. Has your physician ever treated you for drinking?   Yes   No

19. Do you drink to build up your self-confidence?   Yes   No

20. Have you ever been to a hospital or institution on account of drinking?
    Yes   No

If you have answered yes to any one of these questions, there is a definite warning that you may be an alcoholic. If you have answered yes to any two, the chances are that you are an alcoholic. If you have answered yes to any three or more, you are definitely an alcoholic.

Overcoming Denial and Asking for Help

If you answered no to *all* of the previous questions, you may skip the rest of this chapter. If you answered yes to any single question and you are truly sincere about seeking help for your anger problem, read ahead, then contact one or more of the resources listed at the end of this book, regardless of whether you actually believe you have a drinking problem. Maybe you have a drinking problem, maybe you don't, but making an educational inquiry doesn't automatically mean you are an alcoholic.

It is normal to feel threatened or scared at this point. Self-searching can be very uncomfortable; you may have a lot of unpleasantness locked inside you and protected on the fragile outer edges by denial. Denial is the hundred-foot wall, the largest, most seemingly insurmountable obstacle that always stands between suffering and healing. Subconsciously, or on some level at least, you have probably always known that wall was there. Whether or not you are aware of your wall of denial, you have been trying to dig your way out like a prisoner until you can't dig any more, and then you hit your bottom.

What Is Alcoholism?

Only in recent years has it been discovered that alcoholism, also known as *alcohol dependence,* is actually a chronic and progressive disease, not just maladjustment in character or mental illness, as was previously believed. Alcoholism has become pervasive in our present-day society; it is believed that nearly 13 percent of all Americans have some type of drinking problem (NIAAA 1995), and the number continues to grow larger as more and more people are reaching out for help. The effects of alcoholism are all-encompassing in the devastation and havoc they create in a person's life. Neglect of responsibilities pertaining to family, employment, or school; continually being involved in alcohol-related legal problems; driving while under the influence; and failure or dissolution of previously meaningful friendships and relationships ("burning bridges") have all become recognized as the infamous hallmarks of alcoholic behavior.

Unfortunately, there is no cure for alcohol dependence problems, but there are an infinite number of recovery programs available that offer hope and success. Recovery in the proper sense is considered to be a remission from the disease, but it requires a lifelong commitment to abstinence, restructuring of attitudes and behavior, and adopting a spiritual lifestyle while continually attending recovery meetings.

Remember that alcoholism is a disease. Simply stopping your alcohol use will not correct the problem, nor will it correct any anger problems you are trying to deal with either. In fact, sudden cessation of alcohol use may actually increase your tendency toward aggression as well as create serious physical problems, which may include the sudden onset of withdrawal symptoms. You should seek professional help before undergoing a self-prescribed detoxification program. The Resources section at the end of this book includes national organizations; for local or regional programs, consult your Yellow Pages, directory assistance, or the Internet. In a crisis situation, or if you just feel like you need to talk to someone for support or advice regarding an alcohol problem, there are twenty-four-hour Alcoholics Anonymous hotline numbers that are usually staffed by experienced volunteers and have proven to be an invaluable and sometimes even lifesaving resource for all those who want it, even at 4:00 A.M. These services are local or sometimes regional and again can be found by directory assistance or the Internet under the heading "alcoholism." The sooner you seek help, the closer you will be to recovery and restoring normalcy and happiness in your life. Take the step.

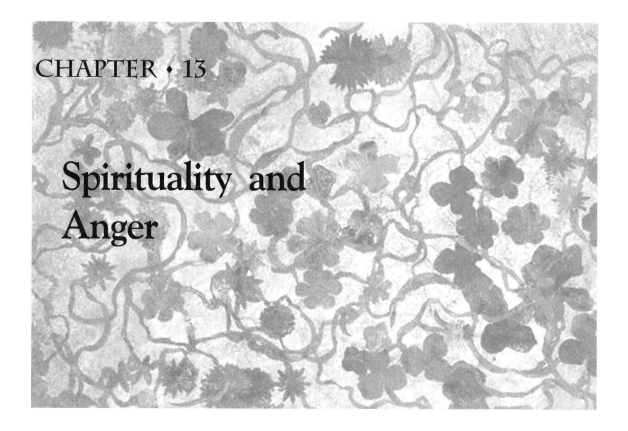

CHAPTER · 13

Spirituality and Anger

SPIRITUALITY IS neither synonymous with nor equal to religion; it does not lend itself easily to a definition in words. Among other things, it is a belief in God or some other higher power, a sense of well-being, and a feeling of actuality. For many people who are trying to overcome major problems or obstacles, spirituality has become a necessary part of their daily routine, because it is a way to make your life a lot easier. The Buddhists believe that life is meant for suffering, a negative plane of existence where we are constantly tested and given hard lessons to learn. Consider all the major traumas you have been through, the very things you are angry at: death or loss of a loved one, family and relationship problems, disease or physical handicaps. These life lessons invariably arrive in very ugly packages. If we deal with these situations with the right action or intent using spiritual guidelines, the blow will be softened, we will suffer less, and we will become stronger and better able to deal with life tragedies as well as those situations that constantly incite our anger. This is not a recipe for total bliss and absolute happiness, only a means to a better end.

This chapter will narrow down the large topic of spirituality to focus on the aspects that are going to help you let go of your anger. The language of "letting go" is entirely and completely spiritual, and absolutely nothing else—short of major tranquilizers and shock therapy—will ever come close to being as successful in helping you reach this goal.

The Serenity Prayer

At the end of every anger management group that I lead, the women and I hold hands in a circle and recite the Serenity Prayer. For building a sense of spirituality, this ritual has proven an important tool for dealing with any problem, especially anger issues, and is used worldwide in twelve-step recovery programs.

> *God, grant me the serenity*
> *To accept the things I cannot change,*
> *The courage to change the things I can,*
> *And the wisdom to know the difference.*

You may immediately be turned off by the mention of God or prayer, but rest assured, I am not asking you to go to church, join a cult, or set up an altar in your basement for relentless, ongoing worship. Spirituality is not religion, but to gain a true spiritual sense, understand that you must surrender your will and acknowledge your defeat in all previous attempts at control, because you never really were in control. In order to surrender, you must personally believe in a higher power, someone or something you feel comfortable turning your life over to. In the past, women have been known to use nonreligious icons, pagan symbols, their pets, and even doorknobs as a higher power. You don't even have to give your higher power a name. Just begin by believing that one exists and that it is ready to take over for you the minute you surrender.

Let's take a closer look at the Serenity Prayer concepts of acceptance, courage, and wisdom.

ACCEPTANCE

It's easier to accept than it is to fight. But learning to live a life of acceptance means accepting people and situations you can't change and focusing on yourself, closely watching your own attitudes and behavior. Stop playing the victim. Acceptance is about moving onward and not getting stuck in the mud of life or dwelling on anger by complaining, blaming, resenting, and faultfinding.

COURAGE

Change requires courage. The familiar, even when it's painful, offers a sense of security in contrast to the fear of the unknown. Recovery from anger issues involves change, and change involves risk. It requires a lot of courage to ask for help, and even more courage to talk about yourself in a group setting. By making yourself open and vulnerable to others, you can free your repressed emotions and feel a sense of catharsis. However, the process of healing is sometimes like pouring a stinging antiseptic on an infected wound. It is painful at the time, but afterward, the pain will be diminished and the wound will heal better.

WISDOM

When anger ties up our emotions, we develop erroneous ideas. Our biggest lie to ourselves—and to everyone else—is that we are never at fault for our own anger. When we are upset or angry, we tend to blame the person or situation for causing our anger. We admit no responsibility for our own part and cling to a sense of self-righteousness.

It's your fault I got angry. I told you to stop and leave me alone—you know how I get, you wanted me to blow up. This is your fault!
      —Sally

Wisdom means properly identifying and then owning your behavior. Change may come later as a part of your surrender and acceptance, but the wisdom is in realizing that people or situations cannot make you angry. You make yourself angry as a response to a situation. You have a choice; the problem is not outside, but rather inside, and even if the other person does have an anger problem too, the only person you can change is yourself.

Incorporating the ideas of acceptance, courage, and wisdom, you could sum up the Serenity Prayer as follows:

I cannot change the past.
I can change my attitude about it.
I have the ability to choose how I feel and act.

Choose a specific situation in your life that you feel resentful, angry, or upset about.

1. Name the particular situation that you cannot change (for example, your childhood, your partner's behavior, or the state of the economy).

. . . .

. . . .

. . . .

. . . .

. . . .

2. List what can change about this particular situation (for example, your attitude or your response to this situation).

. . . .

. . . .

. . . .

. . . .

. . . .

3. List other conflicts you are encountering now. Describe aspects you can and cannot change about these situations (for example, you can change where you work; you cannot change your boss).

. . . .

. . . .

. . . .

. . . .

. . . .

❧

Surrender

The first step to solving any problem is to admit that it even exists. The exercises in this book are meant to help you identify your anger problems; understand your anger triggers, behavior patterns, and resentments; and begin to remedy your reactions. The next step involves spirituality, self-searching, and an inventory of your life. The end purpose is to facilitate a safe outward expression for the anger living inside of you.

A mere academic understanding of your problem is a step in the right direction, of course, but without the willingness, courage, and patience needed to effectively deal with your anger problem, you will remain intellectually detached. That is, you will be an expert on your own behavioral history, knowing everything about your own anger, but remaining unable or unwilling to do the time-consuming and oftentimes painful work that is required for true change and healing—to surrender, accept, and then let go.

To surrender means to get down on your knees, figuratively or perhaps even literally, and realize that the situation will never change until the direction of your life changes. To surrender is to relinquish your self-will and control over your life. To surrender is to accept the fact that you are a person who has suffered misdirected guidance and let self-will run riot, believing *I can do it myself, I don't need anybody's help.* Surrendering means accepting the fact that your life has become unmanageable, as twelve-step recovery programs say. To surrender is to accept that you cannot change the situations happening outside of you, only how you choose you respond to them, and finally, to accept outside help from people and programs. Get down on your knees, and get out of your head.

When we finally get to the turning point of surrender, it is usually because of great suffering or loss. If we hadn't suffered or lost anything, would we have a motive to change our behavior? Changing attitudes and behavior is not an easy task, especially if we don't have a reason why we should do so in the first place. In the following pages are some exercises that will help you understand why you have arrived at this turning point.

What have been the consequences of your anger?

For each category below, list at least three examples of how anger has hurt you or others.

Physical health:

. . . .

. . . .

. . . .

. . . .

Employment:

. . . .

. . . .

. . . .

. . . .

Relationships:

. . . .

. . . .

. . . .

. . . .

Money:

. . . .

. . . .

. . . .

. . . .

Spirituality (or morals or ethics):

. . . .

. . . .

. . . .

Mental anguish:

. . . .

. . . .

. . . .

Other:

. . . .

. . . .

. . . .

❖

Moral Inventory

How clear is your conscience? You need to look at both your present and your past to see how you have behaved in this respect. This self-searching is not about confession, or about repentance for your sins, or even about beating yourself up and thinking you are a bad person, because you are not. Simply stated, taking an inventory of how your anger has hurt others is part of making a commitment to change. You can't change your behavior in the future if you don't look at your actions and begin to understand your patterns of wrongdoings.

Step four of the twelve-step recovery program is to make "a searching and fearless moral inventory" of yourself (*Alcoholics Anonymous* 1976, 59). This is considered to be one of the most powerful tools of self-discovery and reconciliation. The following exercise was created with the fourth step in mind, and it is designed to help you start acknowledging the mistakes you have made. This gives you an opportunity to start holding yourself accountable for your anger issues. If you do not hold yourself accountable for your actions, you cannot expect to change your actions. This exercise will not be easy to do. In fact, doing a thorough job will almost certainly bring up painful feelings such as fear, shame, and regret. Honesty is absolutely essential; if you minimize or deny your part in this inventory, then it is doubtful that you will receive any appreciable benefit from completing it. Answer each question in a factual way, without blaming others. This will require taking a good hard look at your behavior.

This exercise requires you to acknowledge how your anger has hurt others without mentioning how they have mistreated you.

1. Make a list of everyone whom your anger has harmed in some way.

. . . .

. . . .

. . . .

. . . .

. . . .

. . . .

2. Looking at the above list of names, think about the particular incidents that harmed each person. List each incident below by type.

Emotional harm

. . . .

. . . .

. . . .

Physical harm

. . . .

. . . .

. . . .

3. Choose three incidents from the list you just made, and describe what you really wanted from others when you used angry behavior.

What I did:

. . . .

What I really wanted:

. . . .

What I did:

· ·

What I really wanted:

· ·

What I did:

· ·

What I really wanted:

· ·

4. List at least three examples of how you kept your repressed anger secret.

· ·

· ·

· ·

· ·

· ·

5. Write an honest expression of at least three feelings you have about mistreating others. Giving lip service to your feelings is not good enough.

· ·

· ·

· ·

· ·

· ·

· ·

6. List at least seven examples of your excuses, attitudes, or beliefs about your behavior, and label
   each one an excuse, attitude, or belief.

. . . .

. . . .

. . . .

. . . .

. . . .

. . . .

. . . .

. . . .

. . . .

♣

Learning Gratitude

It's hard to feel grateful sometimes, especially when you think about all the stuff you've been through. Yet, gratitude is an important tool in developing your spirituality. Nowadays it seems the natural human condition is to always see the cup half empty, never half full. We take what we have for granted. We are materialistic consumers, not spiritual beings. We justify our materialism by pointing out everything bad and negative in our society. How are we supposed to feel grateful? So we keep trying to fill that dark, empty void inside us with anything from the outside. But satisfaction is only temporary; you must "feed the void" again, and again, and again. In between feedings, you feel empty, lost, and angry. Sound familiar?

Only by adapting our attitudes to the challenging situations at hand will we ever learn our spiritual lessons and adapt our responses in kind. Adaptation allows us to lessen the suffering we feel, to loosen the grip that anger has upon us, and to feed that black hole with the proper nourishment it needs. Adapting is a method of permanently changing our attitude to one of forgiveness, gratitude, and eventually serenity. In this way, we learn to flow with the turbulent current rather than swim against it. The end result is that we expend less emotional energy to deal with life on life's terms; we become happier people.

List five things that you are thankful for in your life. Continue this daily gratitude list in your journal, and make five entries per day. Do this first thing in the morning, so that you can start the day off in a positive state of mind.

1. . . . .

2. . . . .

3. . . . .

4. . . . .

5. . . . .

Now try to imagine how your life would be without the item on your gratitude list above. List here the negative consequences if you didn't have the items above.

For example, suppose you wrote *I have a good car.* Below, you might write *If I didn't have a car that runs well, I would not be able to get to work. There is no public transportation, and I don't have any money to buy a new car.*

1. . . . .

. . . .

2. . . . .

. . . .

3. . . . .

. . . .

4. . . . .

. . . .

5. . . . .

. . . .

Narrative Therapy

Narrative therapy, or storytelling, is a powerful healing method that uses aspects of self-searching, spirituality, and safe expression of anger. This concept originated in the Jungian school of thought and was later adapted and specifically applied as a powerful tool for healing women's anger in the 1992 writings of Clarissa Pinkola Estes. The act of putting feelings and situations into story form is not only a safe outlet but also a way to unearth fossils buried deep inside. Estes believes that women possess within themselves the ability to heal their rage and anger by seeking a wise and calm healing force in their own psychic territory, thereby putting old obsessive thoughts and feelings to rest. In order to heal, women must understand the power of the spiritual self and seek solutions: What caused this rage, and how can I use it constructively to heal myself? If we look at anger from this Jungian perspective, the outside world may be chaotic and fallen to pieces, while the inside world—the spiritual self, the healer—remains unshaken by external happenings, staying calm and serene while searching for a solution.

By writing your own anger story, you can instill within yourself a creative force to heal your anger, to heal yourself.

Write your responses to each question. If you are working with an anger management group, share your anger story with the other women in the group. This is a powerful exercise when you do it alone, but it is especially powerful when you tell your story to others.

1. What has your life been like? Where do you think your anger problem came from?

. . . .

. . . .

. . . .

. . . .

. . . .

2. What happened? What anger incident or consequence made you decide to buy this workbook or join an anger management group?

. . . .

. . . .

. . . .

. . . .

3. What is your life like now? How have you changed since completing most of this workbook, participating in an anger management group, or completing individual therapy surrounding your anger?

. . . .

. . . .

. . . .

. . . .

. . . .

. . . .

❧

Healing Anger with Forgiveness

Actual healing is accomplished in small increments, usually over a period of months and years. It is not the all-or-nothing transformation many anger management books claim. The idea here is progress, not perfection, so don't despair. Many women have gone through anger recovery and reported life-changing results and immeasurable relief from the burden of anger. When you begin to feel hopeless or unsure about your progress, remember this: you have suffered an entire lifetime of anger, and not even the best therapist or the best anger recovery book can turn you into a saint overnight. It took more than two weeks for you to get this way, so it's certainly going to take more than two weeks to fix it! A serious, ongoing commitment is required to obtain results in any recovery program. Anger is considered a healthy emotion when it's used properly, so don't expect to banish it from your repertoire, never to be seen or felt again. Instead, work toward diminishing the control that anger has over your life and replacing it with something more comforting and less destructive: a sense of serenity.

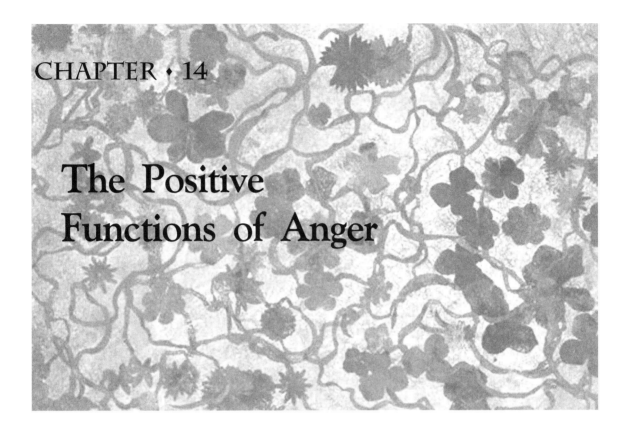

CHAPTER ◆ 14

The Positive Functions of Anger

IN THE anger groups I facilitate, I often hear women say proudly, "I didn't get angry at all this week!" I remind them that not getting angry is not the goal of treatment. On the contrary, not getting angry usually leads to an outburst of anger that was held down for too long. Acknowledging your anger and then expressing it in an appropriate manner is the goal of treatment.

Women often consider anger "bad" because they mistakenly associate it with violence. Anger isn't necessarily good or bad. Anger is an important emotion for women to feel, just like other emotions are. So, again, the goal is not to completely eliminate anger from your life, but to use it as an appropriate response to situations and people. The research and literature on anger agree that anger can be positive for women.

There is no one definition of constructive anger; it depends on the situation and circumstances. Anger serves as a messenger (Potter-Efron and Potter-Efron 1991), as a teacher (Estes 1992), and as a clue that something is wrong (Lerner 1988). Women can use their anger to learn to identify issues (Lerner 1988), gather up their energy to respond to a perceived threat (Person 1993), and discover how to change, grow, and take care of themselves (Estes 1992). Anger can play a positive role in the workplace, too (DiGiuseppe and Tafrate forthcoming).

Anger can also be used as a source of power when targeted against societal or personal injustice. "Imagine what the women's movement would have been like," explains Carol Tavris (1989, 301) "if women had said, 'Guys, it's really unfair, we're nice people and we're human beings too. Won't you just listen to us and give us the vote?'" Much of the progress in the women's rights movement was fueled by the anger of the leaders and demonstrators. My own anger has had many benefits. Upset by the inequality of my salary compared to that of my male coworkers, I decided to further my education. Dismayed by the lack of anger workbooks for women, I found that anger gave me some of the drive to write this book.

Women can express their anger in a useful and positive way through constructive problem solving. Constructive anger expression usually involves both people, not just one person venting at another. In a win-win situation, a woman expresses her anger, and her partner hears her and responds with his or her own thoughts and feelings. If your anger is heard and the misunderstanding is corrected, the situation can usually be corrected. Anger can be constructive, says Tavris (1989, 301), when both people look at the situation as a problem to be solved mutually, not an opportunity for a woman to dump her feelings on another. "The question is not, 'Should I express anger or should I suppress it?' It is, 'What can we do to solve the problem?'"

Constructive Problem Solving

Women with anger problems often need help in developing more positive ways of approaching and solving problem situations. The following strategies will help you approach and deal with problems in a controlled manner, without using your anger destructively. Take time to learn these strategies and practice using them when you are in problem situations.

❧   Make sure you are in a calm state of mind before confronting the problem.

❧   Decide on your goal. Pick only one issue at a time.

❧   Accept responsibility for your own feelings by using I-language.

❧   When bringing up or discussing a problem, always focus upon the other person's behavior (what he or she is doing or not doing) rather than personality. For example, say, "I would like you to become better at being on time" rather than "You're such an unreliable jerk." Emphasize the positive by simply saying what you want rather than saying what you don't want.

❧   Stick to your issue. Don't get sidetracked.

❧   If others disagree with you, remember to listen to their point of view. Restate in your own words what they said.

❧   Be willing to negotiate a solution. Avoid getting into an *I'm right, you're wrong* battle.

❧   Agree on what you have negotiated. Shake on it!

CONSTRUCTIVE PROBLEM-SOLVING CUE CARD

1. Get control of yourself.

    —Breathe—

2. Pick one issue.

3. Use I-language.

4. Ask for the behavior you want.

    —Relax—

5. Stick to your issue.

6. Listen and restate.

    —Breathe—

7. Negotiate.

8. Seal the deal:

I will _____ .

You will _____ .

Keep in mind that change is slow. The important thing is to keep trying and to forgive yourself for lapses or setbacks. Making a commitment to work on anger can only improve your life—and perhaps it already has, if you have been doing the exercises in this book.

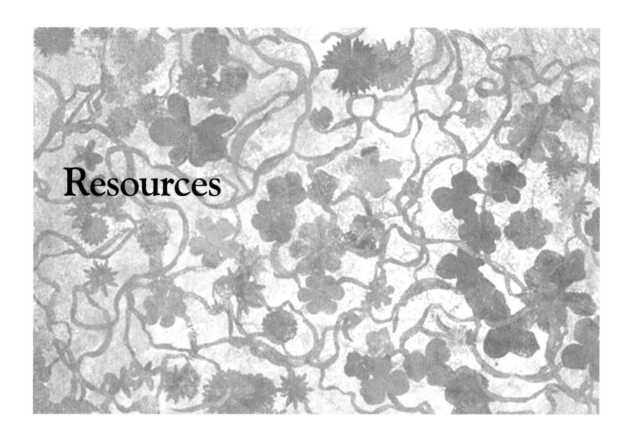

Resources

General Anger Resources

Laura Petracek, Ph.D.
www.angermanagementforwomen.com
Includes training for therapists in how to use this workbook for groups.

Resources for Alcohol Problems

Al-Anon Family Group Headquarters, Inc.
1600 Corporate Landing Parkway
Virginia Beach, VA 23454-5617
Phone: (757) 563-1600
Fax: (757) 563-1655
Web site: www.al-anon.alateen.org

Alcoholics Anonymous (AA) World Services, Inc.
475 Riverside Drive, 11th Floor
New York, NY 10115
Phone: (212) 870-3400
Fax: (212) 870-3003
Web site: www.alcoholics-anonymous.org

National Council on Alcoholism and Drug Dependence, Inc.
20 Exchange Place, Suite 2902
New York, NY 10005
Phone: (212) 269-7797
Fax: (212) 269-7510
Web site: www.ncadd.org

National Institute on Alcohol Abuse and Alcoholism, Scientific Communications Branch
Willco Building, Suite 409
6000 Exchange Boulevard
Bethesda, MD 20892-7003
Phone: (301) 443-3860
Fax: (301) 443-1726
Web site: www.niaaa.nih.gov

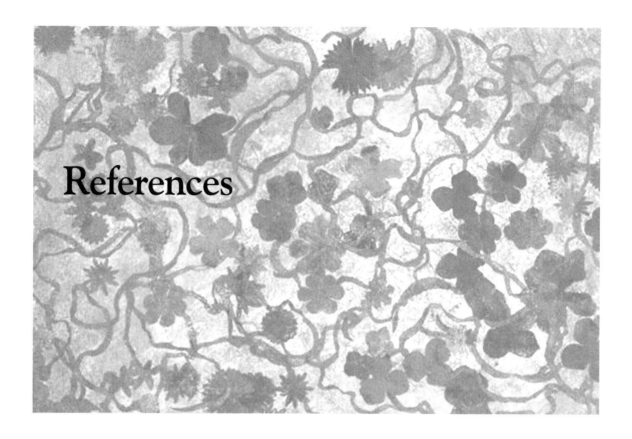

References

Alcoholics Anonymous. 1976. 3rd ed. AA World Services, Inc.

Arnow, Bruce, Justin Kenardy, and W. Stewart Agras. 1992. Binge eating among the obese: A descriptive study. *Journal of Behavioral Medicine* 15(2):155–70.

Barnhill, Julie Ann. 2001. *She's Gonna Blow!* Eugene, Oreg.: Harvest House Publishers.

Bass, Ellen, and Laura Davis. 1988. *The Courage to Heal.* New York: Harper & Row.

Beck, Aaron. 1976. *Cognitive Therapy and the Emotional Disorders.* New York: International Universities Press.

Beck, Aaron, and Gary Emery. 1985. *Anxiety Disorders and Phobias: A Cognitive Perspective.* New York: Basic Books.

Black, Claudia. 1981. *It Will Never Happen to Me.* Denver: MAC Publishing.

Campbell, Anne. 1993. *Men, Women, and Aggression.* New York: Basic Books.

Cox, Deborah, Sally Stabb, and Karin Bruckner. 1999. *Women's Anger: Clinical and Developmental Perspectives.* Philadelphia: Brunner/Mazel.

Crawford, June, Susan Kippax, Jenny Onyx, Una Gault, and Pam Benton. 1992. *Emotion and Gender.* London: Sage Publications.

Deffenbacher, Jerry, Deborah Story, Robert Stark, James Hogg, and Allen Brandon. 1987. Cognitive-relaxation and social skills interventions in the treatment of general anger. *Journal of Counseling Psychology* 34(2):171–76.

DiGiuseppe, Raymond, and Raymond Tafrate. In press. *The Anger Disorder Scale Manual*. Toronto: Multi-Health Systems.

Emerson, Carol, and David Harrison. 1990. Anger and denial as predictors of cardiovascular reactivity in women. *Journal of Psychopathology and Behavioral Assessment* 12(4):271–83.

Estes, Clarissa Pinkola. 1992. *Women Who Run with the Wolves*. New York: Ballantine Books.

Folkman, Susan, and Richard Lazarus. 1980. An analysis of coping in a middle-aged community sample. *Journal of Health and Social Behavior* 21:219–39.

Hamberger, Kevin. 1991. Characteristics and context of women arrested for domestic violence: Context and implications. *Marital Violence: Theoretical and Empirical Perspectives* (May):Paper presented at conference.

Lane, Mary Rockwood, and Michael Samuels. 1998. *Creative Healing: How to Heal Yourself by Tapping Your Hidden Creativity*. San Francisco: HarperSan Francisco.

Lauersen, Niels, and Eileen Stukane. 1983. *PMS, Premenstrual Syndrome and You: Next Month Can Be Different*. New York: Simon & Schuster.

Lerner, Harriet Goldhor. 1985. *The Dance of Anger*. New York: Harper & Row.

Lerner, Harriet Goldhor. 1988. *Women in Therapy: Devaluation, Anger, Aggression, Depression, Self-Sacrifice, Mothering, Mother Blaming, Self-Betrayal, Sex-Role Stereotypes, Dependency, Work and Success Inhibitions*. Northvale, N.J.: J. Aronson.

Modcrin-McCarthy, Mary Anne, and Jane Tollett. 1993. Unhealthy, unfit, and too angry to care? In *Women and Anger*, edited by Sandra Thomas. New York: Springer Publishing.

Munhall, Patricia. 1992. Women's anger and its meanings: A phenomenological perspective. *Health Care for Women International* 14:481–91.

NIAAA. March 17, 1995: NIAAA Releases of Estimates of Alcohol Abuse and Dependence and Alcohol Alert No. 23: *Alcohol and Minorities*.

Person, Ethel Spector. 1993. Introduction to *Rage, Power, and Aggression*, edited by Robert Glick and Steven Roose. New Haven: Yale University Press.

Potter-Efron, Patricia, and Ronald Potter-Efron. 1991. Anger as a treatment concern with alcoholics and affected family members. *Alcoholism Treatment Quarterly* 8(3):31–46.

Russell, Sheryl, and Barbara Shirk. 1993. Women's anger and eating. In *Women and Anger*, edited by Sandra Thomas. New York: Springer Publishing.

Saylor, Margaret, and Gayle Denham. 1993. Women's anger and self-esteem. In *Women and Anger*, edited by Sandra Thomas. New York: Springer Publishing.

Sells, Sam, and Peter Loosen. 2000. Bipolar disorder. In *Current Diagnosis and Treatment in Psychiatry*, edited by Michael Ebert, Peter Loosen, and Barry Nurcombe. New York: Langer Medical Books/McGraw-Hill.

Spielberger, Charles, D. 1988. State-Trait Anger Expression Inventory (STAXI). Lutz, Fla.: Psychological Assessment Resources.

Tangney, June Price, Patricia Wagner, Carey Fletcher, and Richard Gramzow. 1992. Shamed into anger? The relation of shame and guilt to anger and self-reported aggression. *Journal of Personality and Social Psychology* 62(4):669.

Tannen, Deborah. 1990. *You Just Don't Understand: Women and Men in Conversation*. New York: Morrow.

Tavris, Carol. 1989. *Anger: The Misunderstood Emotion.* Revised edition. New York: Simon & Schuster.

Thomas, Sandra. 1993. Anger and its manifestations in women. In *Women and Anger,* edited by Sandra Thomas. New York: Springer Publishing.

Thomas, Sandra, and Madge Donnellan. 1993. Stress, role responsibilities, social support, and anger. In *Women and Anger,* edited by Sandra Thomas. New York: Springer Publishing.

Thomas, Sandra, and Cheryl Jefferson. 1996. *Use Your Anger: A Woman's Guide to Empowerment.* New York: Pocket Books.

Weisinger, Hendrie. 1985. *Dr. Weisinger's Anger Work-Out Book.* New York: Quill.

Woodman, Marion. 1980. *The Owl Was a Baker's Daughter: Obesity, Anorexia Nervosa, and the Repressed Feminine.* Toronto: Inner City Books.

Laura J. Petracek, Ph.D., is assistant professor of clinical psychology at National University in Sacramento, CA. She maintains a private practice in San Francisco and is a certified treatment provider for the San Francisco Department of Probation. She is a member of the American Psychological Association, the National Association of Alcohol and Drug Addiction Counselors, and the Nation Association of Social Workers.

Foreword writer Sandra Thomas, Ph.D., RN, FAAN, is director of the doctoral program at the University of Tennessee College of Nursing in Knoxville, TN. She has studied women's anger since 1989. Initial findings from her women's anger study—the first large-scale investigation of the emotion in American women—were published in the 1993 book *Women and Anger*, which received extensive coverage from national press and television programs.

Some Other
New Harbinger Titles

Talk to Me, Item 3317 $12.95

Romantic Intelligence, Item 3309 $15.95

Transformational Divorce, Item 3414 $13.95

The Rape Recovery Handbook, Item 3376 $15.95

Eating Mindfully, Item 3503 $13.95

Sex Talk, Item 2868 $12.95

Everyday Adventures for the Soul, Item 2981 $11.95

A Woman's Addiction Workbook, Item 2973 $18.95

The Daughter-In-Law's Survival Guide, Item 2817 $12.95

PMDD, Item 2833 $13.95

The Vulvodynia Survival Guide, Item 2914 $15.95

Love Tune-Ups, Item 2744 $10.95

The Deepest Blue, Item 2531 $13.95

The 50 Best Ways to Simplify Your Life, Item 2558 $11.95

Brave New You, Item 2590 $13.95

Loving Your Teenage Daughter, Item 2620 $14.95

The Hidden Feelings of Motherhood, Item 2485 $14.95

The Woman's Book of Sleep, Item 2493 $14.95

Pregnancy Stories, Item 2361 $14.95

The Women's Guide to Total Self-Esteem, Item 2418 $13.95

Thinking Pregnant, Item 2302 $13.95

The Conscious Bride, Item 2132 $12.95

Juicy Tomatoes, Item 2175 $13.95

Facing 30, Item 1500 $12.95

The Money Mystique, Item 2221 $13.95

High on Stress, Item 1101 $13.95

Perimenopause, 2nd edition, Item 2345 $16.95

The Infertility Survival Guide, Item 2477 $16.95

Call **toll free, 1-800-748-6273,** or log on to our online bookstore at **www.newharbinger.com** to order. Have your Visa or Mastercard number ready. Or send a check for the titles you want to New Harbinger Publications, Inc., 5674 Shattuck Ave., Oakland, CA 94609. Include $4.50 for the first book and 75¢ for each additional book, to cover shipping and handling. (California residents please include appropriate sales tax.) Allow two to five weeks for delivery.

Prices subject to change without notice.

After the Breakup, 1764 $13.95